J. Carman Sr.

W9-BBW-084

Emergency First Response

Primary Care and Secondary Care

Participant Manual

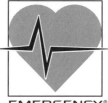

EMERGENCY®
first response

EMERGENCY°
first response

Emergency First Response

This Participant Manual belongs to_____

Mailing Address_____

City_____State/Province _____

Zip/Postal Code_____Country_____

Phone Number_____

Instructor Statement:

I certify that this person has completed the following Emergency First Response course requirements and indicated recommended skills.

❑ **Primary Care (CPR)**

Instructor Signature_____ Number_____

Completion Date_____

    ❑ **Recommended Skill – Automated External Defibrillator (AED) Use**

    Instructor Signature_____ Number_____

    Completion Date_____

    ❑ **Recommended Skill – Conscious Choking Adult**

    Instructor Signature_____ Number_____

    Completion Date_____

    ❑ **Recommended Skill – Emergency Oxygen Use**

    Instructor Signature_____ Number_____

    Completion Date_____

❑ **Secondary Care (First Aid)**

Instructor Signature_____ Number_____

Completion Date_____

Emergency First Response
Primary Care and Secondary Care Participant Manual

©Emergency First Response Corp., 2005

All rights reserved.

Produced by DSAT (Diving Science and Technology Corp.) for Emergency First Response, Corp.

No reproduction of this book is allowed without the express written permission of the publisher.

Published and distributed by Emergency First Response, Corp.

30151 Tomas Street • Rancho Santa Margarita, CA 92688

Printed in the U.S.A. • Product No. 70091 (Rev. 1/05) Version 2.0

For More Information

For more information about Emergency First Response, Corp., courses, products and emergency care go to www.emergencyfirstresponse.com.

Patient Care Standards

Emergency First Response Primary Care (CPR) and Secondary Care (First Aid) follow emergency considerations and protocols from the consensus view of the Basic Life Support (BLS) Working Group of the International Liaison Committee on Resuscitation (ILCOR). ILCOR is an international standards group representing many of the world's major resuscitation organizations. A source authority for the development of content material in the Emergency First Response program is Guidelines 2000 for Cardiopulmonary Resuscitation and Emergency Cardiovascular Care, International Consensus on Science, *Circulation*, 2000; Vol. 102 (suppl I); ©2000 American Heart Association®, Inc.

Acknowledgements

International Medical Review
Phil Bryson, MBChB, DCH, DRCOG, MRCGP
Medical Director
Diving Disease Research Centre, UK

Des Gorman, BSc, MBChB, FAFOM, PhD
Head - Occupational Medicine
School of Medicine, University of Auckland
Auckland, New Zealand

Jan Risberg, M.D. PhD
Begen, Norway

Brian Smith, M.D.
Mountain West Anesthesia
Utah, USA

Technical Consultant
Jon Sowers, EMT
Training Director
Emergency Medical Training, Inc.

International Development, Writing, Consultation & Review
Bob Wohlers, Brad Smith, Julie Taylor Sanders, Lori Bachelor-Smith, Karl Shreeves, Dana Stewart, Drew Richardson, Suzanne Pleydell, Mike Holme, Brigit Jager, Henrik Nimb, Jean-Claude Monachon, Pascal Dietrich, Trond Skaare.

Design, Typography & Production
Janet Klendworth, Joy Zuehls, Greg Beatty, Joe De La Torre

About this Manual

The *Emergency First Response Participant Manual* has three sections

- **Section One – Independent Study Workbook**
- **Section Two – Skills Workbook**
- **Section Three – Emergency Reference**

Section One provides you with foundational information specific to Emergency Responder care. By reading the background information in this section, you'll better understand why your role as an Emergency First Responder is so important to those who need emergency care.

Section Two applies to skill development portion of your Emergency First Response course. Under your Emergency First Response Instructor's supervision, you'll use this step-by-step workbook to guide you through a practice session for each of the course's skills.

Section Three provides a quick emergency care reference to use after you complete your Emergency First Response course. This section includes emergency care reference for:

- Primary Care – Rescue Breathing and CPR for Adults, Children and Infants
- Assembling a First Aid Kit
- Injury First Aid – Dislocations, fractures, cuts, scrapes, bruises, dental injuries, strains, sprains, eye injuries and electrical injuries
- Temperature-Related Injuries – Burns, hypothermia, frostbite, heat stroke and heat exhaustion
- Illness First Aid – Heart attack, stroke, diabetic problems, seizures, allergic reactions, poisoning, venomous bites and stings

One
Independent
Study

Contents

Introduction

Someone cuts his finger in a kitchen. At a gym, an older gentleman collapses from a heart attack. During a sporting event, a young boy faints from standing too long. Two automobiles collide, seriously injuring the occupants. A youngster floats motionless, face down in a swimming pool. A diner at the next table chokes on food, unable to breathe.

It happens every day. Some of these people just need a helping hand while others will die or suffer serious permanent injury if not immediately attended to. Many things separate those who live and escape serious disability from those who die or suffer long after their misfortune: the individual's fitness and health, the severity of the initial incident, the distance from medical care and often, just plain luck. No one can control these variables.

But there's one variable you *can* control when you're on the scene of any medical emergency: *You*. Often, life versus death or complete recovery versus long-term disability lies with a layperson first responder providing care between the emergency's onset and the arrival of professional medical personnel. If you are there, you can provide that care. *You* can be an Emergency Responder. As a layperson, you can't guarantee that a patient will live or fully recover — there's too much beyond anyone's control

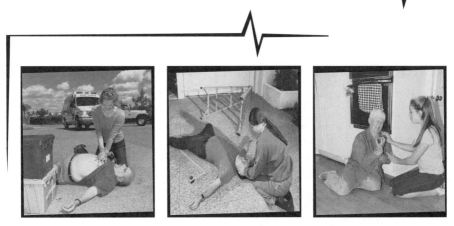

You can be an Emergency Responder. And you'll learn to apply first responder care following the same priorities used by medical professionals.

— but you can feel confident that given the circumstances, everything that could be done will be done.

If you're not familiar with emergency care procedures, it can seem intimidating and complex. What do you do? For that matter, how do you know what to do first? Such questions may appear overwhelming, but actually, they're not. If you can remember "ABCD'S," you'll know what to do. This is because no matter what the nature of a medical emergency, you follow the same steps in the same order, providing basic care based on what you find (see the next page, "The ABCD'S of Emergency Care"). In the Emergency First Response Primary Care (CPR) and Secondary Care (First Aid) courses, you'll learn that ABCD'S prompt you to follow the necessary steps in the right order, so you do the right things at the right time. You'll learn to apply first responder care following the same priorities used by medical professionals.

The ABCD'S of Emergency Care

Emergency First Response Primary Care (CPR) teaches you the steps and techniques for handling life threatening emergencies. You'll learn how to apply the ABCD'S to a patient's *lifeline*. The *lifeline* illustration helps you remember what to do and in what order to provide emergency care. Visualize the *lifeline* illustration as you assist someone in need. Once you reach the end of the *Lifeline* you return to "A" and continue to monitor a patient's *lifeline*.

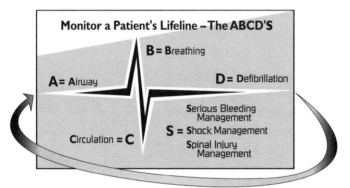

Monitor a Patient's Lifeline – The ABCD'S

B = Breathing

A = Airway   **D** = Defibrillation

Serious Bleeding Management
S = Shock Management
Circulation = **C**   Spinal Injury Management

The ABCD'S of primary care are:

A = Assess Scene, Alert EMS and Airway Open. You assess the scene for safety, call the Emergency Medical Service and open the patient's airway.

B = Breathing. Check the patient's Breathing and if necessary, begin rescue Breathing

C = Circulation. Check the patient for signs of circulation and if necessary, begin Chest Compressions.

D = Defibrillation.

S = Serious bleeding management; Shock management; Spinal injury management

Course Structure

This manual and the *Emergency First Response Video* provide the study tools for two courses — Emergency First Response Primary Care (CPR) and Emergency First Response Secondary Care (First Aid). Your instructor may conduct these courses separately or together.

The Eight Skills Learned in Emergency First Response Primary Care (CPR)

- Scene Assessment
- Barrier Use
- Primary Assessment
- Rescue Breathing
- One Rescuer, Adult CPR
- Serious Bleeding Management
- Shock Management
- Spinal Injury Management
- Recommended Skill – Automated External Defibrillator (AED) Use
- Recommended Skill – Conscious Choking Adult
- Recommended Skill – Emergency Oxygen Use

The Four Skills Learned in Emergency First Response Secondary Care (First Aid)

- Injury Assessment

- Illness Assessment

- Bandaging

- Splinting for Dislocations and Fractures

Emergency First Response Primary Care (CPR) teaches you the steps and techniques for handling life threatening emergencies. In it, you'll learn eight skills for aiding patients who aren't breathing, have no heartbeat, may have a spinal injury, may be in shock or who may have serious bleeding. You'll learn how to apply the ABCD'S to a patient's *lifeline*, so that you provide the patient with every possible chance of survival in the face of the most serious emergencies.

Emergency First Response Secondary Care (First Aid) teaches you what to do when Emergency Medical Services are either delayed or unavailable. This course also teaches you how to provide first aid for patients with conditions that aren't life threatening. You'll learn to apply the ABCD'S so that you can be sure there's no imminent threat to the patient's life while you provide care that reassures, eases pain and reduces the risk of further harm.

For both courses, you'll begin by reading the Independent Study section of this manual and watching

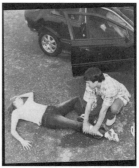

Emergency First Response Primary Care (CPR) teaches you the steps and techniques for handling life threatening emergencies.

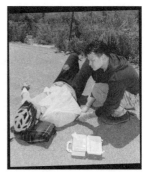

Emergency First Response Secondary Care (First Aid) teaches you what to do when Emergency Medical Services are either delayed or unavailable.

the *Emergency First Response Video*. This gives you the basic information about why each skill is important and how to do it. Then you'll practice the skill with your instructor so that you become capable and comfortable with it. After you've learned all of the skills in each course, your instructor will stage mock emergencies for you and your classmates. During these scenarios, you'll practice applying your skills and learn to adapt what you've learned to circumstances like you might find in real life. You'll find that the emphasis is on learning the skills so that you're comfortable using them.

BEGIN HERE

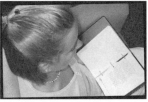

*Read the Independent Study portion
of this Participant Manual.*

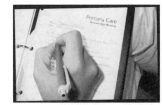

*Complete the Knowledge Review at
the end of the independent study
portion of your Participant Manual.*

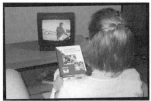

*Watch your Emergency First
Response Video.*

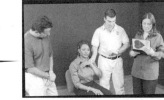

*Attend the Skill Development session
organized by your Emergency First
Response Instructor.*

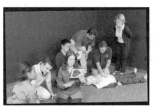

*Complete the Scenario Practice with
your Emergency First Response
Instructor.*

Learning Tips

Here are a few pointers to help you get the most out of the Emergency First Response Primary Care (CPR) and Secondary Care (First Aid) courses.

1. **Don't focus on perfection**. A common misconception with emergency care is that the smallest error will hurt or kill a patient. This is seldom true. Your instructor will make sure you understand what's critical and what's not. When someone focuses on perfection, there's a tendency to do nothing in a real emergency because that person fears not doing everything "perfectly." Don't get caught in that trap — it's not hard to provide *adequate* aid, and adequate aid provided is always better than perfect aid withheld.

2. **Don't be intimidated.** You're learning something new, so don't be surprised if you're not immediately comfortable with a skill or need some guidance. So what? If you already knew how to do it, you wouldn't be there. Mistakes aren't a problem — they're an important part of learning.

3. **Have fun.** That may sound odd given the seriousness of what you're learning, but the truth is, you'll learn more and learn faster if you and your classmates keep things light. Polite humor and light jests are normal in this kind of learning. But, be sensitive and aware that others taking the course with you may have been involved in a situation similar to what you're practicing. You can have fun without seeming insensitive or uncaring about human suffering.

4. **Be decisive and then act.** There's more than one right answer. When you practice the scenarios, you'll find that circumstances don't always give you a clear direction in

exactly how to best apply the ABCD'S. Don't worry — this is exactly why you're doing the mock emergencies. Decide how to apply your training and then do it. It may not be the only way, and later, you may think of a different way that you would have liked better. That's fine for learning, but it doesn't make the way you did it wrong. Never forget that *adequate aid provided is better than perfect aid withheld.*

5. **It all comes back.** When you're practicing the scenarios, you may notice that as you follow the steps within the ABCD'S, things you "forgot" come back to you — not necessarily smoothly at first, but adequately so that you're capable of providing emergency care. Remember that feeling. If you're ever faced with a real emergency and have doubts about remembering what to do, recall this feeling. You can trust that the ABCD'S will bring back what you need to know. *Adequate aid provided is better than perfect aid withheld.*

6. **Complete all your independent study prior to class.** In most situations, your Emergency First Response Instructor will expect you to come to the Skill Development and Scenario Practice session having read all of your *Emergency First Response Participant Manual* and watched the entire *Emergency First Response Video.* Doing so will streamline your learning by allowing you to focus on skill development with your instructor. Begin by scanning a section, read through its *study questions,* then read the section. At the end of the independent study material, you will find one Knowledge Review for each course. Complete the Knowledge Review and bring it to class along with your participant manual.

Who May Enroll In Each Course And What Are The Prerequisites?

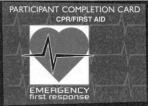

Anyone of any age may enroll in the Emergency First Response Primary Care (CPR) course. The course is performance-based, meaning that as long as you can meet each of the stated objectives and complete the necessary skills to the satisfaction of your instructor, you can receive a course completion card.

To enroll in the Emergency First Response Secondary Care (First Aid) course, you need only complete the Primary Care (CPR) course. Or, if you're currently CPR trained from another qualified training organization, you can enroll directly in the Emergency First Response Secondary Care (First Aid) course with a quick review by your instructor. Examples of other qualified CPR training organizations include: American Heart Association, Red Cross, American Safety and Health Institute, Cruz Roja de Mexico, Deutsches Rotes Kreuz, MEDIC FIRST AID, INC®., Queensland Ambulance Service, South African Red Cross Society and St. John's Ambulance. There may be others that qualify; check with your instructor.

Helping Others in Need

Study Questions

- Why is time critical when someone needs emergency care?

- Why should you assist someone who needs emergency care?

- What are five reasons people hesitate to provide emergency care to a patient – even if they are trained in CPR and first aid?

If you encounter someone who needs primary emergency care and you've assessed the scene for your own personal safety (more on this later), you should render assistance immediately – even seconds count. The chances of successful resuscitation diminish with time. When a person has no heartbeat and is not breathing, irreversible brain damage can occur within minutes. Many medical emergencies, like sudden cardiac arrest, require the secondary assistance of Emergency Medical Service personnel. Get them on the scene fast - seconds count. It is typically best to alert the Emergency Medical Service first, before rendering emergency care (more on this later).

Besides providing an act of kindness toward a fellow human being in need, there are three basic reasons for assisting someone who needs emergency care:

1. You can save or restore a patient's life.

2. You can help reduce a patient's recovery time; either in the hospital or at home.

3. You can make the difference between a patient having a temporary or lifelong disability.

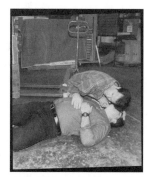

When someone is in need of emergency care, you should render assistance immediately – even seconds count.

1.11

Some individuals, even when CPR and first aid trained, hesitate to provide emergency care to those in need. This is understandable and there are legitimate concerns on the part of Emergency Responders when helping those with injuries and illnesses. The five most common reasons why people hesitate to provide emergency care are:

1. **Anxiety**.

   People may hesitate due to general nervousness or anxiousness. This is a perfectly normal reaction when helping those in need. However, as it's been emphasized, trust your training. Use the ABCD'S prompt to follow the necessary steps in the right order, so you do the right things at the right time.

2. **Guilt**.

   People may hesitate when thinking about how they might feel if the patient doesn't recover after delivering first aid. Once again, remember that as a layperson, you can't guarantee that a patient will live or fully recover — there's too much beyond anyone's control. However, you *can* have confidence that given the circumstances, everything that can be done *will* be done.

3. **Fear of imperfect performance**.

   People may hesitate because they feel they cannot properly help an injured or ill person. It is seldom true that the smallest error will hurt or kill a patient. During this course, you will learn what's critical and what's not. If you focus on perfection, you'll have a tendency to do nothing in a real emergency. Don't get caught in that trap —it's not hard to provide adequate care, and *adequate* aid provided is always better than perfect aid withheld.

4. **Responsibility**.

People may hesitate because they are afraid of being sued. In general, the fear of being sued should not stop Emergency Responders from providing emergency care. In many regions of the world, Good Samaritan laws have been put in place to encourage people to come to the aid of others. More on this in a moment.

5. **Fear of infection**.

People may hesitate because they are afraid of being infected by the person they are assisting. Keep in mind that 70 percent of all CPR is performed in the home or for a loved one or friend. In these cases, risk of infection is low and fear of infection should not cause you to withhold CPR or emergency care. Regardless, the actual risk of disease transmission during CPR is quite small.

Good Samaritan Laws

Good Samaritan laws (or related, local laws) are enacted to encourage people to come to the aid of others. In general, they protect individuals who voluntarily offer assistance to those in need. They are created to provide immunity against liability.

Often, a Good Samaritan law imposes no legal duty to help a stranger in need. However, local laws may vary on this point and in some areas people are required to provide aid. There may not be Good Samaritan laws in your local area. It would be wise to determine the extent and use of Good Samaritan laws in your local area. Your Emergency First Response Instructor may be able to provide you with information about Good Samaritan laws in your local region.

There are four ways you should act to be protected by Good Samaritan laws. They are:

1. Only provide care that is within the scope of your training as an Emergency Responder.

2. Act in good faith.

3. Do not be reckless or negligent.

4. Act as a prudent person would.

Study Questions

- What is a Good Samaritan law?

- In general, what are the four ways you should act to be protected by most Good Samaritan laws?

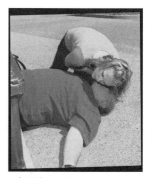

Good Samaritan laws are enacted to encourage people to come to the aid of others.

Chain of Survival

The Chain of Survival illustrates the seven links of patient care. The first three links or actions within the Chain of Survival involve you, the Emergency Responder. All remaining links involve Emergency Medical Service personnel or medical professionals.

Study Question

- What are the Chain of Survival's seven links and which three involve an Emergency Responder?

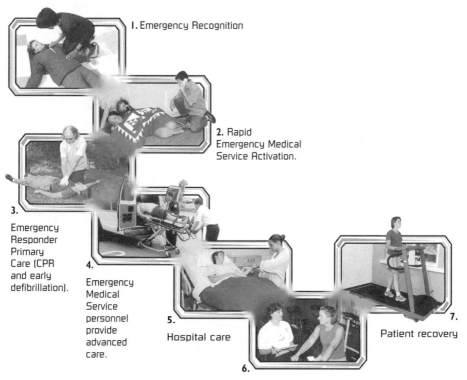

1. Emergency Recognition

2. Rapid Emergency Medical Service Activation.

3. Emergency Responder Primary Care (CPR and early defibrillation).

4. Emergency Medical Service personnel provide advanced care.

5. Hospital care

6. Rehabilitation

7. Patient recovery

Emergency Recognition

As an Emergency Responder you must first recognize that an emergency exists. Once you've determined that an emergency exists, evaluate the scene to determine if it is safe for you to assist the patient. Proper scene assessment is a skill you'll learn in the Emergency First Response Primary Care (CPR) course.

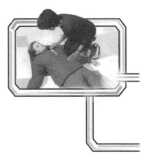

Rapid Emergency Medical Service Activation

For a patient with a life threatening problem, you must rapidly activate the Emergency Medical Service in your local area. This is the *Call First* concept. More on this to come.

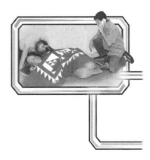

Emergency Responder Primary Care (CPR and early defibrillation)

A person who is not breathing and has no heartbeat needs CPR immediately. CPR is a skill you will learn in the Emergency First Response Primary Care (CPR) course. Early CPR is the best treatment for cardiac arrest until the arrival of Emergency Medical Service personnel. A recommended skill you may be taught in this course is Automated External Defibrillator (AEDs) Use. An AED is key to reviving *an adult* patient suffering from a cardiac emergency involving ventricular fibrillation (twitching heart).

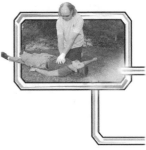

In some countries, however, use of AEDs is reserved for Emergency Medical Service personnel. More on AEDs later.

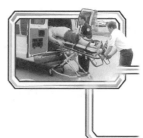

Emergency Medical Service Personnel Provide Advanced Care

Emergency Medical Service personnel can provide advanced patient care such as artificial airways, oxygen, the use of cardiac drugs and even defibrillation when AED's are unavailable or may not be used by Emergency Responders in a local area.

To complete the Chain of Survival, patients move from hospital care to rehabilitation and then to patient recovery.

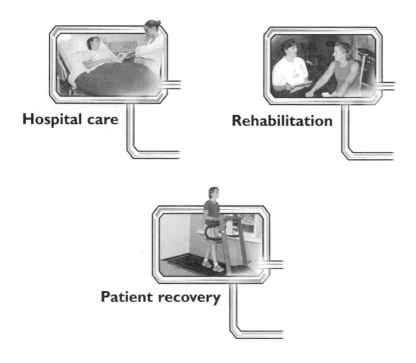

Hospital care

Rehabilitation

Patient recovery

Activating the Emergency Medical Service – Call First

Study Questions

- Why is it important to activate an Emergency Medical Service immediately?

- When should you activate the Emergency Medical Service once you find an unresponsive adult or child who needs emergency care?

If you encounter an individual in need of emergency care for a life threatening problem, it is important to activate your local Emergency Medical Service immediately, even prior to CPR. Doing so increases the patient's chances of survival through early advanced care such as defibrillation, breathing tubes, oxygen and the use of cardiac drugs. Further, the Emergency Medical Services trained dispatcher may be able to assist you in providing emergency care. This is the *Call First* approach to primary care.

Call First means that once you've established unresponsiveness of an adult patient, you *immediately* call an ambulance or activate your local Emergency Medical Service. If help is available, direct others to activate the Emergency Medical Service. When you ask others to call, be specific with your instructions and single out one individual if a crowd is present.

There are some exceptions to the *Call First* approach and local protocol does vary. In the following cases, you'd provide approximately one minute of emergency care prior to activating Emergency Medical Services:

- Submerged child or adult.

- An adult patient suspected of drug overdose.

- An adult patient in arrest due to a serious traumatic injury.

When in doubt however, always use the *call first* approach.

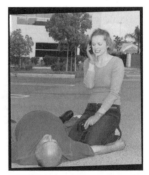

Call first *means that once you've established unresponsiveness of an adult patient, you immediately call an ambulance or activate your local Emergency Medical Service.*

Asking a Patient for Permission to Help

When an injured or ill responsive adult needs emergency care, ask permission before you assist the person. This also acts to reassure the patient, noting that you are trained appropriately. Say, "Hello? My name is _____. I'm an Emergency Responder. May I help you?" If the patient agrees or doesn't respond, proceed with emergency care. If a responsive adult becomes unconscious, most laws assume implied permission – meaning you can proceed with emergency care. You should check the laws in your region.

If a responsive, injured or ill adult refuses emergency care, you do not force it on the person. If possible, talk with the individual and monitor the patient's condition by observation without providing actual care.

Study Questions

- How do you ask for permission to help a patient?

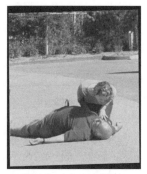

When an injured or ill responsive adult needs emergency care, ask permission before you assist the person. Say, "Hello? My name is _____. I'm an Emergency Responder. May I help you?"

The Emotional Aspects of Being an Emergency Responder

Study Questions

- Why should you never fear harming a patient when performing CPR on an individual whose heart has stopped?

- Why is CPR no guarantee that the patient's heart will restart?

- How can you care for yourself as an Emergency Responder after you've provided emergency care in stressful situations?

Helping another person in need is satisfying and feels good. Depending on the circumstances, however, it may also produce a certain amount of stress and some fearfulness. In most cases a little stress may actually assist you when helping others by preparing you physically and mentally.

CPR and some types of first aid are inherently emotional activities. However, as an Emergency Responder you should never *fear* harming a patient when performing CPR on an individual whose heart has stopped. Why? Simply put – if a patient's heart has stopped you cannot make the person worse. A person with no breathing and no heartbeat is already in the worst state of health. Regardless of how you perform CPR, you cannot make the patient worse than when you first found the individual. You don't need to fear providing CPR rescue breaths and chest compressions. Perform CPR to the best of your ability. Trust your training. Before actually performing CPR, take a moment to relax, then step forward and help. If your efforts to revive the person do not succeed, focus on the fact that you tried your best.

Don't worry about doing something wrong – just

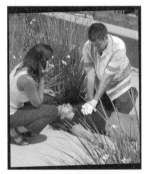

CPR and some types of first aid are inherently emotional activities. However, as an Emergency Responder you should never fear harming a patient when performing CPR on an individual whose heart has stopped.

help. As an Emergency Responder, use your skills to assist others in need. Perform the skills as best you can. As you'll learn a bit later, CPR helps support a patient by forcing oxygen-rich blood from the heart to vital body organs. It's a temporary measure that can extend the window of opportunity for the patient to be revived.

But CPR is no guarantee that the patient's heart will restart. First of all, even with CPR the patient's heart doesn't restart most of the time. Second, there's very little relationship between CPR technique and a patient's heart restarting – so don't worry about your technique. For the most part, layperson CPR is as effective as CPR performed by medical professionals. This means that you can never know if providing CPR would have made a difference unless you step forward and help. If you provide CPR and the patient's heart doesn't restart when Emergency Medical Service personnel arrive, don't second-guess yourself. You did everything humanly possible. But, if you could have provided CPR and didn't, you may spend the rest of your life wondering if helping could have made a difference. Don't hesitate – trust your training.

Providing emergency care to those in need can be emotional. You may have elevated physical and emotional stress after providing emergency care. If you do, try the following:

- Try to relax after the incident. Lower your heartbeat and blood pressure by resting or walking slowly. Relaxing will reduce elevated adrenaline produced by your body to help you through the stress of providing emergency care.

- Avoid stimuli such as caffeine, nicotine or alcohol.

- Talk about the incident to others. Sharing your experience with others helps in processing thoughts and emotions, therefore reducing stress and anxiety. Talk can be a healing medicine.

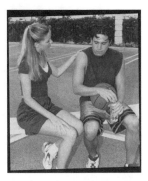

- If you experience physical or emotional problems such as prolonged depression, sleeping disorders, persistent anxiety or eating disorders, seek the help of a health care professional.

- Spend time with others. Reach out – people care.

Keeping Your Skills Fresh

Study Questions

- Why should you practice primary care skills after the course is over?

- How can you practice and refresh your skills?

When this course is completed, make it a point to practice your primary care skills from time to time. When not used or practiced, all skills deteriorate over time. CPR and first aid skills can begin to deteriorate as soon as six months after initial training.

Hopefully, you won't have to use your emergency skills in an actual situation. But if you don't, you will then need to practice your skills to keep them fresh and properly sequenced. You can practice and refresh your skills on your own by:

- Reviewing your *Emergency First Response Video*. Also, glance through this Participant Manual.

- Role-playing scenarios with your family members or friends.

- Walking through the CPR sequence using a pillow or appropriately sized stuffed bag.

- You can also practice monitoring a patient's *lifeline*.

An easy and effective way to practice and fine-tune your emergency care skills is by enrolling in an Emergency First Response refresher. During the refresher, you'll practice by completing the Skill Development portion of an Emergency First Response course with an

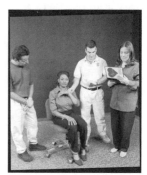

An easy and effective way to practice and fine-tune your emergency care skills is by enrolling in an Emergency First Response refresher.

Emergency First Response Instructor. After completing the refresher, you'll be issued a new Emergency First Response completion card. It's a good idea to take a refresher program at least every 24 months to keep your skills and completion card current.

Leading a Healthy Lifestyle

Study Questions

- What four ways can you keep your own heart healthy and avoid coronary heart disease?

- How can you lead a healthy lifestyle?

In many countries, more men and women die from coronary heart disease each year than from all other causes of death *combined*, including cancer and AIDS. It is fitting to discuss how *you* can reduce your own risk of coronary heart disease and lead a healthy lifestyle. Reducing your risk will also help you be a more fit Emergency Responder. Here are four ways you can reduce your risk of heart disease:

- Avoid exposure to cigarette smoke.

- Reduce stress.

- Eat a diet low in saturated fat and cholesterol.

- Exercise regularly.

Also, if you have high blood pressure or diabetes, keep up with the treatment procedures agreed upon with your doctor. Both high blood pressure and diabetes are risk factors for heart disease.

There are other ways to lead an all-around healthy lifestyle. Consider the following:

- Enjoy living. Don't merely focus on ways to avoid dying.

- Learn to relax, but don't be lethargic.

- Manage stress. Don't merely focus on how to avoid it.

- Live in the world more fully. Don't withdraw from it.

- Take care of yourself, so you are able to function effectively as an Emergency Responder.

Protecting Yourself Against Bloodborne Pathogens

Study Questions

- What three blood-borne pathogens are of greatest concern to Emergency Responders?

- As an Emergency Responder, what four ways can you protect yourself against bloodborne pathogens?

- As an Emergency Responder what general rule may help you avoid infection by bloodborne pathogens?

Infections (viruses, bacteria or other microorganisms) carried by the blood are called bloodborne pathogens. The three *bloodborne pathogens* of greatest concern to Emergency Responders are:

- Hepatitis C virus

- Hepatitis B virus

- Human immunodeficiency virus (HIV)

As an Emergency Responder, there are four ways you can protect yourself against bloodborne pathogens when assisting those in need of emergency care:

- Use gloves.

- Use ventilation masks or face shields when giving mouth-to-mouth rescue breathing.

- Use eye or face shields; including eye glasses or sunglasses, goggles and face masks.

- Always wash your hands or any other area with antibacterial soap and water after exposure. Scrub vigorously, creating lots of lather. If water is not available, use antibacterial wipes or soap-less, antibacterial liquids.

As a general rule, always place a barrier between you and any moist or wet substance originating from a patient. All blood and body fluid should be considered potentially infectious. Take precautions to protect yourself against them.

Fear of disease transmission is a common reason why laypersons trained in CPR avoid action. It is important to note, however, there has never been a recorded case of an injured or ill person infecting a first aid provider using a barrier device. To date, no emergency care provider has ever contracted HIV or hepatitis through rescue breathing.

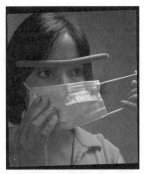

Use of barriers when providing emergency care can protect you against bloodborne pathogens.

Recognizing Life Threatening Problems

When you witness a serious car accident or watch someone take a bad fall, it's reasonable to assume the patient will have life threatening injuries. Even if you don't see it occur, many accident scenes clearly point to medical emergencies.

Unfortunately, not all life threatening emergencies are so obvious. Some serious conditions occur due to illness or subtle accidents. Sometimes the patient's symptoms come on quickly and other times the patient gets progressively worse over time. Because time is critical, as you've already learned, you need to be able to recognize all life threatening conditions and then provide appropriate emergency medical care.

Heart Attack

A heart attack occurs when blood flow to part of the patient's heart is stopped or greatly reduced.

Heart attack patients commonly complain of chest pain and an uncomfortable pressure or squeezing. This usually lasts for more than a few minutes, or goes away and comes back. The pain is sometimes described as an ache, or feeling similar to heartburn or

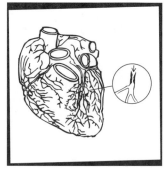

With restricted blood flow, part of the heart muscle begins to die.

indigestion. Pain may spread to the shoulders, neck or arms. Patients may also complain of nausea, shortness of breath and dizziness or lightheadedness. They may sweat or faint.

Often, heart attack patients deny that anything is seriously wrong. This is especially true when symptoms are mild or go away temporarily. If you suspect a heart attack, do not delay in calling EMS or transporting the patient to a medical facility. The longer the heart goes without adequate blood flow, the more permanent damage is likely to occur.

Cardiac Arrest

When a heart artery becomes blocked and the heart stops receiving oxygen, it may begin to quiver – called *ventricular fibrillation* – or just stop beating. This is called cardiac arrest. Although cardiac arrest is most often caused by heart disease or heart defects, it can occur any time regular heart rhythms are disturbed.

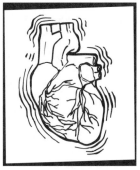

Ventricular fibrillation

There are two ways to recognize cardiac arrest. First, the patient does not respond when you speak to or touch him. Second, the patient does not have signs of circulation – no movement, breathing or coughing. Beginning CPR quickly and providing defibrillation as quickly as possible are critical to patient survival.

Stroke

A stroke occurs when a blood vessel is blocked or ruptures in the patient's brain. Blockage or rupture deprives the brain of oxygen and causes cell death. Signs, symptoms and damage depend on which part of the brain is affected. Five signs and symptoms may indicate stroke:

1. Numbness, paralysis or weakness of face, arm or leg

2. Speech difficulties

3. Facial droop

4. Unexplained headaches

5. Sudden blurred or decreased vision in one eye or both.

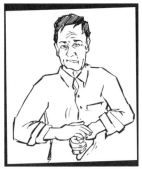

Early recognition and treatment of stroke helps minimize damage to the patient's brain.

Some strokes are mild and last for only a few minutes while others are serious and debilitating. If you suspect a stroke, do not delay in calling EMS or transporting the patient to a medical facility. Mild strokes often precede more serious strokes making immediate medical care crucial.

Complete Airway Obstruction

Complete airway obstruction usually results when a patient chokes on food, although any object placed in the mouth could end up blocking the patient's airway.

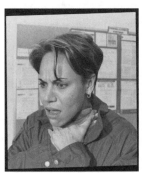

The universal signal for "I am choking."

Recognizing airway obstruction is important because the patient can't speak. Patients also tend to become embarrassed and try to leave the area.

You may suspect choking if a patient grasps or clutches the neck or throat area. By asking the patient what's wrong, you can determine if the patient can speak, is breathing or is able to cough. A patient with a complete airway obstruction may become unconscious if the airway is not cleared quickly.

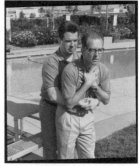

During skill development, you may learn to help dislodge the obstruction and care for a choking patient.

Primary Care Definitions

Primary means *first in a series or sequence;* most important. Assessment is an *evaluation* or an *appraisal.* Primary assessment is your *first evaluation* of an injured or ill person.

During skill development, you'll practice the steps for conducting a primary assessment. These steps help you check for life threatening conditions that need immediate attention. Because attending to life threatening conditions is most important, or primary, to caring for a patient, the action you take based upon your primary assessment is called *primary care.*

Study Questions

- What are Primary Assessment and Primary Care?

- What are the ABCD'S of the *lifeline*?

- What is meant by continually monitor and treat a patient's *lifeline*?

- How do you activate the Emergency Medical Service in your area?

ABCD'S of the *Lifeline*

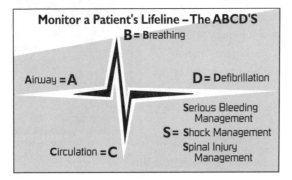

Monitor a Patient's Lifeline – The ABCD'S

B = Breathing

Airway = **A**

D = Defibrillation

Serious Bleeding
Management
S = Shock Management
Spinal Injury
Management

Circulation = **C**

To help you remember the proper sequence of emergency primary care, think:

A = Assess the scene, **A**lert EMS and **A**irway open

B = **B**reathing check and rescue **B**reathing

C = **C**irculation or **C**hest **C**ompressions

D = **D**efibrillation, either by EMS or by an Automated **E**xternal **D**efibrillator

S = **S**erious bleeding management; **S**hock management; **S**pinal injury management

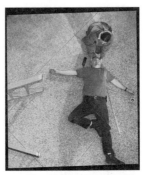

You check for life threatening conditions and follow an important sequence to provide care.

As you'll learn in your skill development session, one of the first things you do when approaching an injured or ill patient is assess the scene. This allows you to decide if the area is safe for you and the patient. It also provides clues about the patient's condition and prompts you to call Emergency Medical Service (EMS).

Once you've judged that it's safe to assist the patient, you begin with a primary assessment following the

ABCD'S in sequence – **A**irway, **B**reathing, **C**irculation, **D**efibrillation, plus **S**erious bleeding management, **S**hock management, and **S**pinal injury management. (You'll read more about these steps and practice each skill with your instructor soon.)

If you find that the patient isn't breathing, you begin rescue breaths. If the patient has no heartbeat, you begin CPR and continue until relieved by EMS personnel. If you find that the patient has no life threatening conditions, but still needs professional medical care, you continue to monitor and treat the patient using the ABCD'S while waiting for EMS. This is what is meant by *continually monitor and treat a patient's lifeline.* The phrase helps you to remember proper primary care sequencing.

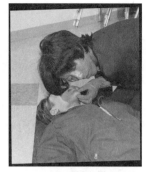

Monitor a patient's lifeline using ABCD'S.

Follow the ABCD'S

Choose the correct sequence of care by numbering the actions (1 to 8) below based on this scenario:
You find a patient lying on the road next to his damaged bicycle. He is unconscious and has no heartbeat. Blood is oozing from around a fence post that is impaled in his leg. After assessing the scene and putting on gloves, you should:

_____ Begin rescue breathing using a barrier

_____ Provide defibrillation using an Automated External Defibrillator - AED

_____ Alert EMS

_____ Check for signs of circulation

__1a__ Open the airway

__3__ Begin CPR (chest compressions)

__2a__ Check for breathing

__5__ Apply pressure to the bleeding leg

Correct Sequence: 1. Alert EMS, 2. Open the airway, 3. Check for breathing, 4. Begin rescue breathing using a barrier, 5. Check for signs of circulation, 6. Begin CPR, 7. Use an AED. 8. You would only attend to the bleeding leg if the patient started breathing and regained a heartbeat. Otherwise, you would continue CPR until relieved by EMS.

Emergency Medical Service

As shown by the Chain of Survival, the extent of care provided by Emergency Responders is limited. One of the most important things you can do to assist a patient with life threatening injuries is to quickly activate the Emergency Medical Service (EMS).

Make sure you know the local phone number and any local protocols involved in calling EMS. It's a good idea to have contact information posted near your home and work phones. Also, discuss procedures with your family and coworkers to ensure that everyone knows how to call for help.

During skill development, you'll practice activating EMS by simulating calls or directing bystanders to summon help. This will reinforce how and when to alert EMS.

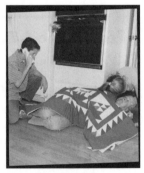

Time is critical – everyone should know how to alert EMS.

Primary Care ABCD'S

Airway and Breathing

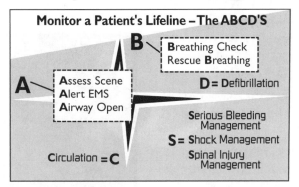

Monitor a Patient's Lifeline – The ABCD'S

B — Breathing Check / Rescue Breathing

A — Assess Scene / Alert EMS / Airway Open

D = Defibrillation

Serious Bleeding Management

S = Shock Management

Spinal Injury Management

Circulation = **C**

Study Questions

- How do you determine if a patient is not breathing during a primary assessment?

- How does rescue breathing work?

- How do you determine if a patient's heart is not beating during a primary assessment?

- What do you do if you don't detect a patient's heartbeat?

- What does CPR stand for, what is it and how does it work?

Besides **A**lerting EMS, the A in the ABCD'S directs you to open the patient's **A**irway. You need to do this because in an unconscious patient, the tongue often falls back and blocks the airway. You may use the head tilt-chin lift

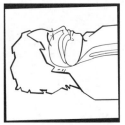

In an unconscious patient, the tongue often falls back and blocks the airway.

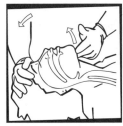

Use the head tilt-chin lift method of opening a blocked airway.

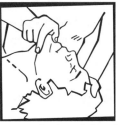

Another technique of hand placement for head tilt-chin lift.

method when there is no evidence of a neck or spinal injury or just the chin lift if a neck injury is suspected. You'll learn both these methods during skill development. With either method, be cautious when handling the patient's head and neck.

With the airway open, you look, listen and feel for **B**reathing. This is part of the B in the ABCD'S. Begin by placing your ear over the patient's nose and mouth. Look toward the patient's chest and see if it rises and falls. Listen for signs of breathing. Feel for the patient's breath on your ear. Your ear is very sensitive, so if the patient is breathing, even lightly, you'll probably feel it. You may also gently place your hand on the patient's chest to feel if it rises and falls.

If you don't detect breathing, you provide rescue **B**reaths – the second part of the B in ABCD'S. By blowing air into the patient's lungs, you provide oxygen. Your expired breath contains plenty of unused oxygen. The air you take in contains 21 percent oxygen and you use only around five percent. This means your rescue breaths contain a very high level of oxygen – more than enough to support a nonbreathing patient. As long as the patient has a heartbeat, rescue breathing will continue to meet the patient's need for oxygen.

Circulation

After handling the A and B of a primary assessment, you move on to C. This is when you determine if the patient

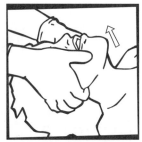

Use the chin lift if a neck injury is suspected.

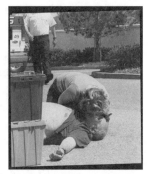

If you don't detect breathing, you provide rescue breaths – the second part of the B in ABCD'S.

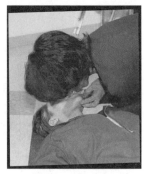

As long as the patient has a heartbeat, rescue breathing will continue to meet the patient's need for oxygen.

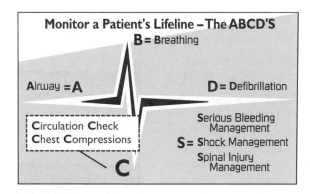

Monitor a Patient's Lifeline – The ABCD'S

B = **B**reathing

Airway = **A**

D = **D**efibrillation

Circulation Check
Chest Compressions

C

Serious Bleeding Management
S = **S**hock Management
Spinal Injury Management

has adequate circulation. When a patient's heart is not beating, there is no circulation of oxygen-rich blood through the body. Checking for circulation is called a Circulation Check.

You conduct a circulation check after providing initial rescue breaths to the unresponsive, nonbreathing patient. With your ear near the patient's mouth, once again look, listen and feel for breathing or coughing. Quickly scan the patient for any signs of movement. If the patient is not breathing, coughing or moving, immediately begin chest compressions or CPR.

Another way to check for a heartbeat is to attempt to locate the patient's carotid pulse. Many people are unable to determine circulation, or the lack of a heartbeat, through a carotid pulse check – especially in older people. If your hands are cold or wet, or if clothing covers the patient's neck, you may have significant difficulty using this method. When in doubt about your abilities to find a carotid pulse, skip this check.

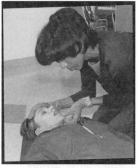

If you can't detect any movement, the patient's heart is not beating.

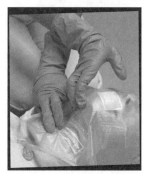

Step 1 – Locate the patient's Adam's apple.

Step 2 – Slide your fingers down into the neck groove and feel for a pulse.

To check for a carotid pulse, start by locating the patient's adam's apple with your index and middle fingers. Slide your fingers down into the groove of the patient's neck on the side closest to you. Take no more than 10 seconds to feel for a heartbeat and make your determination.

CPR

If a patient doesn't have a heartbeat, you begin CPR. CPR stands for *Cardiopulmonary Resuscitation*. It's a skill that combines rescue breathing with manual chest compressions. Providing **C**hest **C**ompressions is the second part of the C in the ABCD'S.

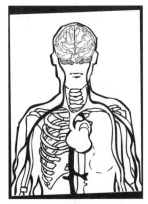

Oxygen-rich blood from the lungs pumps through the heart and is delivered to cells throughout the body.

To understand how CPR benefits a patient, you first must know how the circulatory system works. The heart pumps oxygen-rich blood throughout the body. It also returns the oxygen-poor blood to the lungs for more oxygen. If the heart is beating erratically or not beating at all, rescue breathing alone is ineffective because blood is not circulating.

If a patient's heart has stopped, you substitute the heart's pumping action to circulate blood through the body. Chest compressions force blood from the heart through the arteries and delivers oxygen-rich blood to vital organs. Manual chest compressions deliver no more than one-third of normal blood flow to the body. This means that CPR can only extend the window of opportunity for patient revival for a short time. CPR's primary function is to extend the window of opportunity for

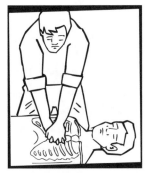

Chest compressions force blood from the heart through the arteries.

patient revival. By performing CPR as an interim procedure, you keep some oxygen rich blood circulating in the patient's body. Even though it's not as efficient as the patient's heart, CPR may support the body until Emergency Medical Service personnel arrive. This is a vital link in the Chain of Survival.

Another reason to consider CPR as an interim step is because it's difficult from an Emergency Responder's perspective to sustain for long periods. Performing CPR can be tiring when performed for an extended period of time. This is why it's so important to activate the Emergency Medical Service immediately.

During skill development, you'll progress from opening the patient's airway and checking for breathing, to providing rescue breaths, to performing CPR.

D is for Defibrillation

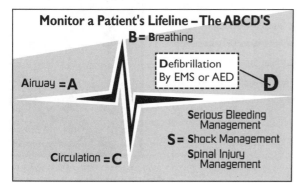

Monitor a Patient's Lifeline – The ABCD'S
B = Breathing
Defibrillation By EMS or AED — D
Airway = A
Serious Bleeding Management
S = Shock Management
Spinal Injury Management
Circulation = C

As discussed, cardiac arrest occurs when something interferes with regular heart rhythms, such as when a blocked artery stops the heart from receiving oxygen. Because a normal heartbeat is triggered by electrical impulses, a malfunction in the system causes the heart to beat erratically or quiver. This erratic beating or quivering is called *ventricular fibrillation. Fibrillation* means to *twitch*.

It is highly unlikely that a heart in ventricular fibrillation will begin beating normally on it's own, even with CPR. To stop the heart from twitching, the erratic impulses must be interrupted. This is accomplished by delivering an electrical shock to the heart. The shock disrupts the abnormal twitching and allows the heart's normal beat to return. Administering an electrical shock is called *defibrillation*.

Early defibrillation is crucial in the Chain of Survival for a patient in cardiac arrest. As an Emergency Responder, you can aid a patient by performing CPR to keep oxygenated blood flowing at a minimal level until Emergency Medical Service personnel defibrillate the patient. Or, you can learn to use an Automated External Defibrillator (AED), which allows you to provide defibrillation to a patient quickly. Because time is critical, being able to use an AED before EMS arrives can significantly increase a patient's chances for survival.

Study Questions

- What is defibrillation and why is it important to a patient whose heart has stopped?

- When a patient's heart is beating erratically or quivering (ventricular fibrillation), what are two ways it can be restored to a normal heart rhythm (defibrillated)?

- What is an Automated External Defibrillator (AED)?

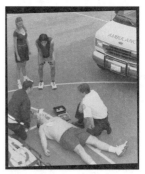

Early defibrillation is necessary to restore a normal heartbeat.

Automated External Defibrillator (AED)

An AED is an easy-to-use, portable machine that automatically delivers a shock to a patient who is not breathing and has no heartbeat. The AED connects to the patient via two chest pads. When the pads are in place, you turn the AED on and its computer analyzes the patient's need for a shock. If it detects a shockable heart rhythm, the machine either independently shocks the patient or directs the Emergency Responder to administer the shock – depending on the AED model.

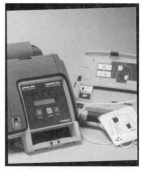

An AED is an easy-to-use, portable machine that automatically delivers a shock to a patient who is not breathing and has no heartbeat.

Because early defibrillation is so important, many businesses, government agencies and institutions are placing AED units in buildings and recreational facilities as well as making them more readily available to law enforcement and rescue personnel.

In some areas AED use is reserved for Emergency Medical Service personnel only. Your instructor may orient you to an AED during skill development.

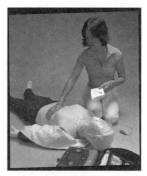

Properly operating an AED is simple with a little training.

The S's

Serious Bleeding, Shock and Spinal Injury

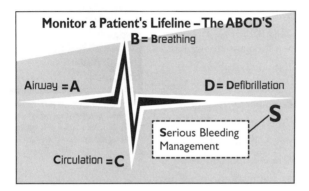

Monitor a Patient's Lifeline – The ABCD'S

B = Breathing

Airway = A

D = Defibrillation

S

Serious Bleeding
Management

Circulation = C

Serious Bleeding Management

Experience tells you that when the skin and underlying tissue is cut, scraped or punctured, there's going to be blood. How much blood flows from the wound and how quickly it leaves the body is what determines whether it's a minor problem or serious bleeding.

The human body contains about six litres/quarts of blood. Rapid loss of just one litre/quart is dangerous and can lead to death. Because serious bleeding is life threatening, you, as an Emergency Responder, need to be able to recognize and manage this during a primary assessment. Serious bleeding management is the first S in the ABCD'S.

Study Questions

- What are the three types of bleeding and how are each identified?

- What is shock, what can cause it and what are the nine indications of shock?

- What does the spinal cord do in the human body and why is it important to protect the spinal cord during primary care?

- What seven indications might signal the need for spinal injury management?

- In what eight circumstances should you always suspect a spinal injury?

- What are two situations where you must move an injured or ill person?

In general, there are three types of bleeding. In an emergency, it's not critical for you to diagnose the exact type of bleeding. However, by knowing the differences, you'll be better able to judge how serious the wound is and how best to manage it. During skill development you'll learn how to control bleeding using direct pressure and pressure points.

Arterial Bleeding

Bright red blood that spurts from a wound in rhythm with the heartbeat. This is the most serious type of bleeding since blood loss occurs very quickly. If a major artery is cut, death can occur within a minute.

Venous Bleeding

Dark red blood steadily flowing from the wound without rhythmic spurts. This bleeding can also be life threatening and must be controlled as quickly as possible.

Capillary Bleeding

Blood slowly oozing from the wound. This slow bleeding may stop on its own or is typically easy to handle with direct pressure.

Any time a patient has serious bleeding, use barriers and activate the Emergency Medical Service immediately and quickly render care to prevent excessive blood loss.

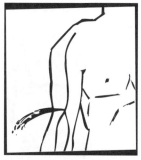

Arterial Bleeding

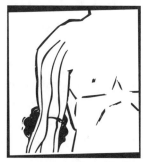

Venous Bleeding

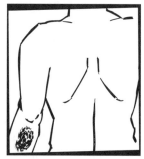

Capillary Bleeding

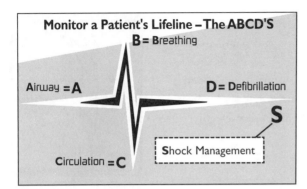

Monitor a Patient's Lifeline – The ABCD'S

B = **B**reathing

Airway = **A**

Circulation = **C**

D = **D**efibrillation

S

Shock Management

Shock Management

Any injury or illness, serious or minor, which stresses the body may result in shock. In reaction to a medical condition, the body pools blood into one or more vital organ. This reduces normal blood flow to other body tissues depriving cells of oxygen. During shock, the body begins to shut down. Shock is a life threatening condition that is easier to prevent from getting worse than it is to treat after it becomes severe. **S**hock management is the second S in the ABCD'S.

During primary assessment and care, you take the first steps to managing shock by dealing with other life threatening conditions. Checking that a patient is breathing, has adequate circulation and is not bleeding profusely helps the patient's body maintain normal blood flow. You render additional care by keeping the patient still and maintaining the patient's body temperature. You may elevate the patient's legs if it won't aggravate another injury. Continuing to monitor the patient's *lifeline* until EMS arrives also contributes to shock management.

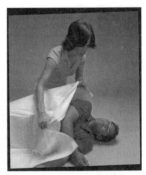

Manage shock by keeping the patient still and maintaining the patient's body temperature.

To identify shock in a patient, look for these nine indications:

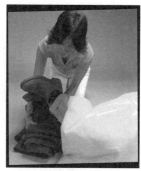

You may also elevate the patient's legs to manage shock.

1. Rapid, weak pulse

2. Pale or bluish tissue color

3. Moist, clammy skin – possibly with shivering

4. Mental confusion, anxiety, restlessness or irritability

5. Altered consciousness

6. Nausea and perhaps vomiting

7. Thirst

8. Lackluster eyes, dazed look

9. Shallow, but rapid, labored breathing

Even if you don't recognize any of these signs and symptoms in a patient, continue to manage for shock when you provide emergency care to an injured or ill patient. Remember, it's better to prevent shock than to let it complicate a patient's condition.

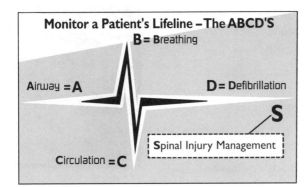

Monitor a Patient's Lifeline – The ABCD'S

B = **B**reathing

Airway = **A**

D = **D**efibrillation

S

Spinal Injury Management

Circulation = **C**

Spinal Injury Management

The spinal cord connects the brain with the rest of the body and organs. Nerve impulses, or messages between the brain and the body travel through the spinal cord. An intact, functioning spinal cord is essential for life.

Vertebrae are a ring of bones surrounding the spinal cord and run from the neck to the lower back. These bones make up the backbone, or spinal column.

A spinal cord injury may result in permanent paralysis or death. The higher up in the spinal column the injury, the more likely it will cause a serious disability. This is why it's so important to guard the head, neck and spine when attending to an injured patient.

Important: **Never move a patient unless absolutely necessary.**

A patient with a severe injury will likely be unable to move. However, a less severe spinal injury will not necessarily keep a patient down. Accident victims often try to get up and move away from the scene. Because an injured

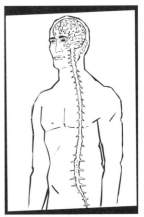

The spinal cord is surrounded by vertebrae that protect it. A serious blow, fall or jolt could cause a break and damage the cord.

spinal cord is fragile, allowing a patient to walk around could turn a minor injury into a permanent disability.

If you suspect a neck or spinal cord injury, keep the patient still and support the head to minimize movement. If you must open the patient's airway, use the chin lift method – do not tilt or move the patient's head. If CPR is necessary and you must position the patient flat on the back, turn the patient as a unit – avoid twisting or jarring the spine.

If you didn't see the injury occur or the circumstances surrounding an injury are not clear, look for these indications that may signal the need for spinal injury management:

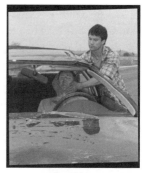

Any time you suspect a head, neck or spine injury, minimize movement.

- You see a change in the patient's consciousness – like fainting.

- The patient has difficulty breathing.

- The patient complains of vision problems.

- When asked, the patient can not move a body part.

- The patient has a headache.

- The patient vomits.

- When walking or sitting, the patient suffers a loss of balance.

- The patient complains of tingling or numbness in hands, fingers and feet or toes.

These are common indications of a back or neck injury, however none may be present even though the patient has an injury. So, regardless of whether these indications are present or not, if you think a person has an injured neck or back, treat it as such.

Spinal injuries generally result from falls or other blows associated with accidents. There may be other incidents that injure the spine, but you should always suspect a spinal injury in these circumstances:

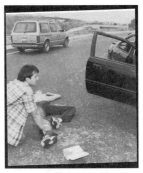

It's always better to assume the patient has a neck or spine injury and not move the patient unless absolutely necessary.

1. Traffic or car accident

2. Being thrown from a motorized vehicle

3. Falling from a height greater than victim's own height

4. Severe blow to the head, neck or back

5. Swimming pool, head-first dive accident

6. Lightning strike

7. Serious impact injury

It's always better to assume the patient has a neck or spine injury and not move the patient unless absolutely necessary. When you approach any patient, handle the patient's head, neck and spine carefully.

When you must move. . .

As just discussed, you should move an injured or ill person only if it's absolutely necessary. This includes circumstances of clear and direct danger to the patient's life, or if emergency care is impossible due to a patient's location or position.

Situations in which you may need to move a patient to give emergency care include:

- Patient is in water.

- Patient is near a burning object or structure that may explode.

- Patient is under an unstable structure that may collapse.

- Patient is on an unstable slope.

- Patient is on a roadway and you can't effectively direct traffic away from patient's location.

Many other situations may apply. You may discuss these with your instructor during skill development while you learn and practice the steps for scene assessment. By taking a moment to assess an accident scene, you help protect yourself from life threatening hazards and prevent the patient from suffering further harm.

During skill development, you'll also practice turning a patient while protecting the neck and spine. This technique for moving a patient is called the log roll. You'll learn to roll a patient by yourself and with the assistance of another Emergency Responder.

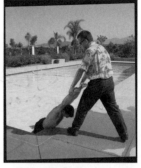

Only move a patient when the location is hazardous or prevents you from providing care.

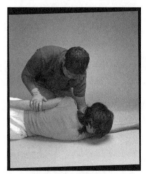

During skill development, you'll also practice turning a patient while protecting the neck and spine.

Primary Care
Knowledge Review

Name: _JLanners Sr_

Date: _4-5-06_

1. When someone needs emergency care, time is critical because: (Check all that apply.)

    ✓ a. It becomes more difficult to administer first aid.

    ✓ b. The chances of successful resuscitation diminish with time.

    ✓ c. When a person has no heartbeat and is not breathing, irreversible brain damage can occur within minutes.

2. From the introductory statements below, which one would you select when asking permission to help a patient? (Place a check by your response.)

    ___ a. I'm a doctor. May I help you?

    ✓ b. Hello? My name is _____, I'm an Emergency Responder. May I help you?

    ___ c. Are you hurt? Where?

3. You should never fear harming a patient when performing CPR on an individual whose heart has stopped because you cannot make the person worse.

    ✓ True

    ___ False

4. As an Emergency Responder what general rule may help you avoid infection by bloodborne pathogens? (Place a check by your response.)

✓ a. Always place a barrier between you and any moist or wet substance originating from a patient.

___ b. Ask the patient not to cough when you are giving him emergency care.

___ c. Have the patient bandage his own bleeding wounds whenever possible.

5. On the lifeline diagram below, list the meaning for each of the letters in the ABCD'S of emergency care.

Monitor a Patient's Lifeline – The ABCD'S

B = _Breathing_

A = _Assess, Airway,_

D = _Defib._

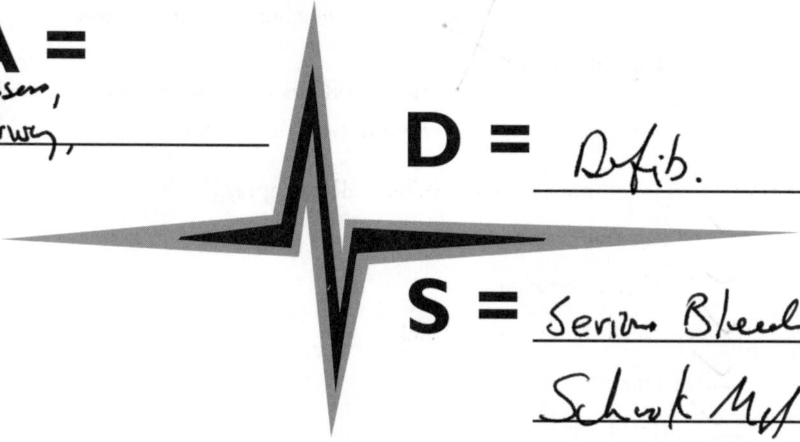

S = _Serious Bleeding_ _Schok Mgt_ _Spinal Injury_

Chest Compression _Circulation_ **= C**

6. How do you activate the Emergency Medical Service in your area?

Phone number:_____

7. Why is defibrillation important to a patient with cardiac arrest? (Place a check by your response.)

____✓ a. Defibrillation disrupts the abnormal twitching of a heart, restoring a normal heartbeat.

____ b. Defibrillation causes the heart to beat erratically.

____ c. It keeps the patient from having to go to the hospital after CPR has been administered.

8. Match the type of bleeding listed below with the description of how each is identified. (Draw a line from the description to the type of bleeding.)

a. Arterial Bleeding

b. Venous Bleeding

c. Capillary Bleeding

• Dark red blood, steadily flowing from a wound without rhythmic spurts.

• Blood slowly oozing from the wound.

Bright red blood that spurts from a wound in rhythm with the heartbeat.

9. What are indications of shock. (Check all that apply.)

____✓ a. Pale or bluish tissue color

____✓ b. Altered consciousness

____✓ c. Lackluster eyes, dazed look

____✓ d. Thirst

____✓ e. Rapid, weak pulse

____ f. Elbow pain

✔ g. Mental confusion, anxiety, restlessness or irritability

___ h. Nausea and perhaps vomiting

✔ i. Moist, clammy skin, perhaps with shivering

___ j. Shallow, but rapid and labored breathing

___ k. Earache

10. In what circumstances should you *always* suspect a spinal injury? (Check all that apply.)

✔ a. Lightning strike

✔ b. Serious impact injury

✔ c. Falling from a height greater than victim's own height

✔ d. Traffic or car accident

✔ e. Being thrown from a motorized vehicle

✔ f. Swimming pool, head-first dive accident

Secondary Care (First Aid)

Introduction

Every day people have mishaps or get sick. Some may be involved in bad accidents or suffer from serious illness, yet remain conscious and responsive. Their conditions may not be immediately life threatening, yet they still need medical care.

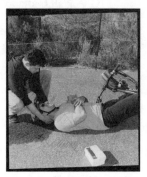

You provide secondary care to an ill or injured patient who is responsive.

Emergency First Response Secondary Care (First Aid) teaches you to assist injured or ill patients by offering first aid and support while waiting for Emergency Medical Service (EMS) personnel. The course prepares you to render emergency care for common medical problems that are not immediately life threatening.

As you learned in your Emergency First Response Primary Care (or other CPR course), any time you approach a patient to provide emergency care, regardless of the injury or illness, you perform a primary assessment and monitor the patient's *lifeline*. During this course, you'll review the ABCD'S – assuring there is no imminent threat to the patient's life – then practice providing care that reassures, eases pain and reduces the risk of further harm.

If EMS is close at hand, you may never need to use the skills in this course. However, if EMS is unavailable or delayed or there is time and distance between the patient and professional medical care, you may need to use your skills to render first aid.

Four Skills of Emergency First Response Secondary Care

- Injury Assessment
- Illness Assessment
- Bandaging
- Splinting for Dislocations and Fractures

Secondary Care
(First Aid)

Definitions

Secondary means *second in a series or sequence.* An assessment is an evaluation or appraisal. Secondary assessment is your second evaluation of an injured or ill person. Once a patient is stabilized during primary care, you attend to the next level of emergency care – *secondary care.* This is the care you provide to a patient with injuries or illnesses that are not immediately life threatening.

During skill development, you'll practice injury assessment that helps you determine the location and extent of all the patient's injuries. You'll also learn the steps for illness assessment that help you identify and report medical problems that affect a patient's health and may aid in treatment. Bandaging wounds, sprains and strains along with splinting dislocations and fractures round out the skills you need to provide secondary care.

Study Questions

- What is a Secondary Assessment and Secondary Care?
- What is the difference between injury and illness?
- What is Assessment First Aid?

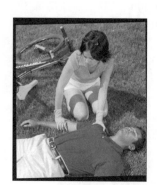

Injury Assessment

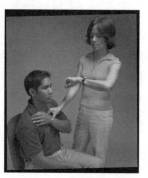

Illness Assessment

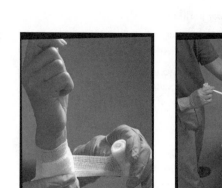

Bandaging

*Splinting for Dislocation
and Fracture*

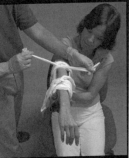

Injury vs. Illness

Throughout this manual, you've read the words injury and illness. When discussing secondary care, it's important to understand exactly what these terms mean.

An injury is defined as physical harm to the body. Examples include:

- Cuts, scrapes and bruises

- Chest wounds

- Head, eye and dental wounds

- Burns

- Dislocations and fractures

- Temperature-related problems – hypothermia, frostbite, heat exhaustion and heat stroke

- Electrical wounds

An illness is an *unhealthy condition of the body*. Illnesses may be caused by preexisting conditions such as allergies, heart disease or diabetes. They may also occur due to external factors such as breathing toxic fumes or ingesting poison. Generally, illnesses are determined by looking for clues or signs that the patient's body is stressed and also by listening to the patient describe symptoms.

Signs and Symptoms

- A sign is something you can *see, hear or feel*.

- For an injury assessment you look for signs such as wounds, bleeding, discolorations, or deformities. You also listen for unusual breathing sounds and feel for swelling or hardness, tissue softness or unusual masses.

- For an illness assessment you look for changes in skin color, breathing rate or patient awareness along with shivering or seizures. You listen for breathing difficulty and you feel the patient's skin temperature and pulse.

- A symptom is something the *patient tells* you is wrong.

- For both injury and illness assessments, the patient may complain of nausea, thirst, dizziness, numbness or pain.

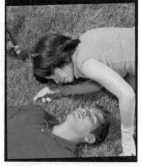

You look, listen and feel for signs.

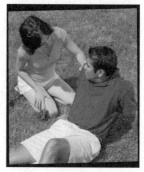

A patient tells you symptoms.

Medical Alert Tags

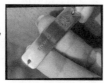

In a medical emergency, information is critical. People with serious medical conditions or severe allergies may wear medical alert tags to provide instant information to Emergency Responders. Usually worn as necklaces, bracelets or other jewelry, these tags may list the patient's

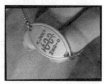

medical problem, medications, allergies and physician, hospital or relative contact numbers.

When a patient is unresponsive or is having difficulty communicating, check for a medical alert tag. It can provide you with the information you need to provide proper care.

What is Normal?

It's difficult to determine if an ill patient's signs are abnormal if you don't know what is "normal." The fact is that what is normal for one patient may be completely abnormal for another. There are "normal" ranges for breathing rate, pulse and skin temperature. However, a patient could be outside the average and still be within a personal "normal" range. This is why it's important when giving information to EMS personnel to avoid using the word *normal* and simply provide measured rates per minute and use other descriptive terminology.

Here are the average ranges that may help guide your assessment:

- The average breathing rate for adults is between 12 and 20 breaths per minute. A patient who takes less than 8 breaths per minute, or more than 24 breaths per minute, probably needs immediate medical care.

- The average pulse rate for adults is between 60-80 beats per minute.

- Average skin temperature is warm and skin should feel dry to the touch.

Assessment First Aid

Assessment first aid is the *treatment of conditions that are not immediately life threatening*, uncovered during either an illness assessment or an injury assessment. For example, applying a bandage to a wound or wrapping a shivering patient in a warm blanket is assessment first aid.

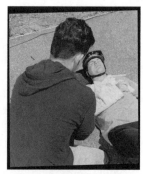

Assessment first aid is the treatment of conditions that are not immediately life threatening.

Although the emphasis of the Emergency First Response Secondary Care (First Aid) course is on rendering emergency care until EMS arrives, you'll find that you may also use your skills to handle common minor medical problems. Cleaning and dressing a child's scraped knee is assessment first aid. Placing a cool compress on a family member's head to relieve flu symptoms is also assessment first aid.

In every situation that involves injury and illness, you'll follow the sequence and steps that you learn and practice in this course. For emergency care and first aid information that is more specific, for example – what to do for a snakebite, use the reference section of your *Emergency First Response Participant Manual*.

Secondary Care
Knowledge Review

Name: _J Lamey Sr_ Date: _4-5-06_

1. Regardless of a patient's injury or illness, you perform a ___b___ assessment and monitor the patient's ___a___. (Place the correct letter in the blank.)

    a. secondary; line of life

    b. primary; *lifeline*

2. Once a patient is stabilized during primary care, you attend to the next level of emergency care - _____.

    a. injury care

    b. secondary care

3. An injury is defined as _Physical bodily han_

4. An illness is defined as _unhealthy condition_.

5. A symptom is: (Place a check by your response.)

    __ a. something the patient tells you is wrong

    __ b. something you can see, hear or feel

6. Assessment first aid is the treatment of conditions that are not immediately _life threatening_.

Two
Skills Workbook

Contents

Primary Care (CPR)

Primary Care Skill # 1
Scene Assessment

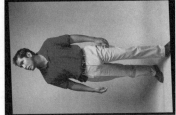

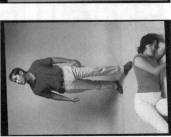

Monitor a Patient's Lifeline – The ABCD'S

B = Breathing

D = Defibrillation

Serious Bleeding
Management

S = Shock Management

Spinal Injury
Management

A

Circulation **= C**

Assess Scene
Alert EMS
Airway Open

Your Goal

Demonstrate the procedures for assessing an emergency scene for safety.

How It's Done
I. STOP – Assess Scene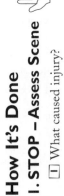

1. What caused injury?

2. Are there any hazards?

3. Can you make a safe approach?

2. THINK – Formulate Safe Action Plan 💡

1. Can you remain safe while helping?
2. What emergency care is needed?
3. How can you activate local EMS?
4. Think about your training and relax.

3. ACT – Alert EMS and Provide Care ✋ 📱

1. Alert EMS.
2. Follow emergency care guidelines.
3. Continue to consider your safety.

Try it ⎍— In your practice group, work through the scene assessment steps for the scenarios on the next two pages. Use steps 1-3 – STOP, THINK and ACT – to assess the scene and form an action plan.

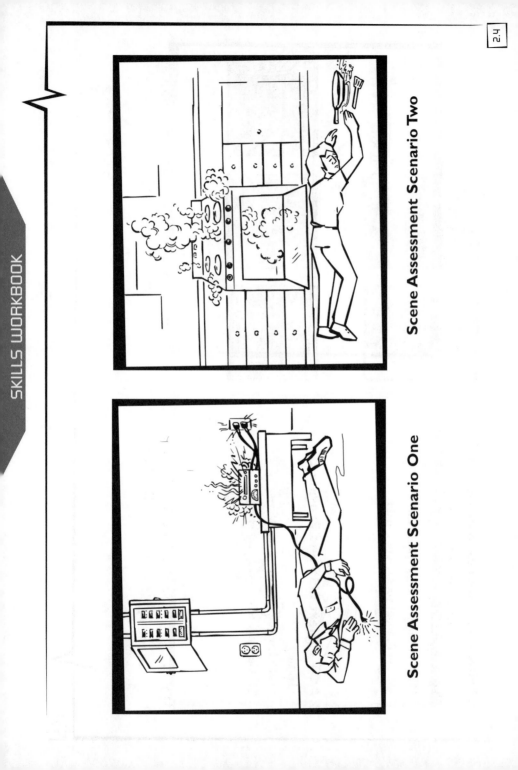

Scene Assessment Scenario Two

Scene Assessment Scenario One

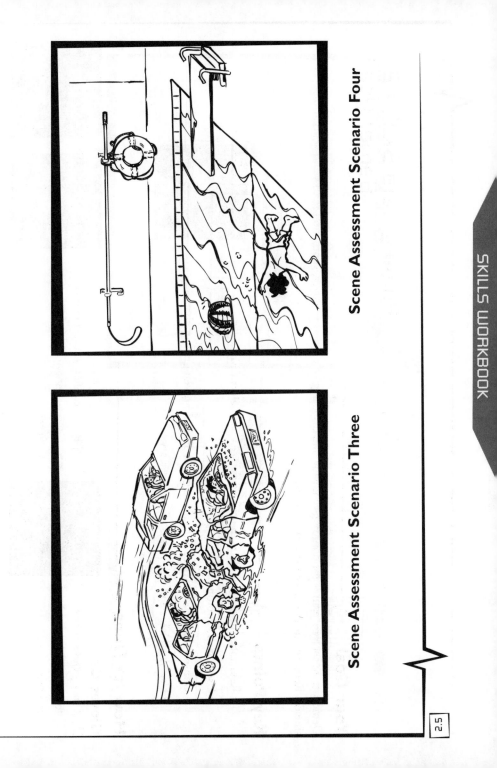

Scene Assessment Scenario Four

Scene Assessment Scenario Three

Primary Care Skill # 2
Barrier Use

Your Goal

Demonstrate the procedures for donning, removing and disposing of barriers – gloves, ventilation shields. Remove gloves without snapping or tearing.

Key Points

- Remember to stop, think, then act – assess scene and alert EMS.
- Use barriers appropriately.
- Consider using more than one pair of gloves around broken glass or sharp objects.
- Use eye shields and face masks when necessary.

How It's Done

Gloves On

1 Quickly check gloves for holes: Blow into gloves and twist closed.

2 Put on carefully to avoid tearing. Consider removing sharp rings on fingers.

☐ Gloves Off

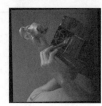

To remove first soiled glove, carefully pinch the outside portion of the glove at wrist. Avoid contact with the outside of the glove. **Be careful not to snap or tear the glove during removal.**

2 Gently roll glove off so that the outside portion is turned inside. Hold the removed glove with the gloved hand.

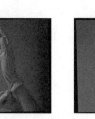
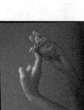

3 To remove remaining glove, place the ungloved hand under the glove at the wrist, next to the skin, and roll off in the same manner. Roll the glove off and around the previously removed glove.

4 Place in biohazard bag for disposal.

Ventilation Barriers

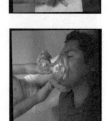

☐ Place ventilation barrier over patient's mouth and/or nose. See photos for placement of different types.

2 Position barrier to allow rescue breaths.

3 Place used disposable ventilation barrier in biohazard bag.

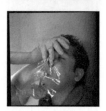

Try It — In your practice group, carefully put on and take off your gloves. Be careful not to tear or snap them as fluids may disperse inappropriately. Also practice placing ventilation barriers on a mannequin as directed by your instructor.

Primary Care Skill # 3
Primary Assessment

Your Goals

Demonstrate how to:

- Perform a patient responsiveness check by giving the Emergency Responder statement.
- Take the *call first* approach and activate the local Emergency Medical Service (EMS) using the correct number.
- Use barriers appropriately.
- Perform a breathing check using the look, listen and feel technique.
- Open a patient's airway using the head tilt-chin lift method when there is no evidence of a neck injury.
- Open a patient's airway using the chin lift method when a neck injury is suspected.
- Place a nonresponsive, breathing patient in the recovery position.

Key Points

- Remember to stop, think, then act – assess scene and alert EMS.
- Use barriers.
- Monitor and treat a patient's *lifeline*.

European Protocol for Activating Emergency Services
The Alert Step for activating EMS (Emergency Service) is completed after checking the patient for breathing.

Monitor a Patient's Lifeline – The ABCD'S

B = Breathing

D = Defibrillation

Serious Bleeding Management
S = Shock Management
Spinal Injury Management

Circulation = **C**

A

Assess Scene
Alert EMS
Airway Open

2.8

How It's Done

Conscious and responsive patient

1 Give responder statement — *Hello? My name is _____. I'm an Emergency Responder, may I help you?* If no response, tap patient on shoulder or arm and ask, *Are you okay?*

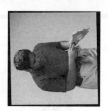

2 If patient responds, it verifies an open airway, breathing and circulation – ABCD. Continue with primary assessment – the S's. Serious bleeding, shock and spinal injury management.

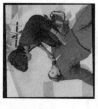

3 Alert EMS.

4 Keep patient still – do not move.

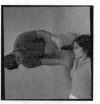

5 Put on barriers

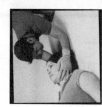

6 Look for serious bleeding – feel for moisture.

7 Treat for shock by keeping the patient comfortable and monitoring ABCD'S.

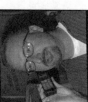

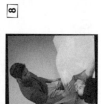

8 Determine if a spinal injury is possible and present. Keep the patient's head, neck and spine immobilized.

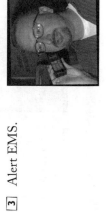

Unresponsive and unconscious patient

1 Give responder statement — *Hello? My name is _____. I'm an Emergency Responder, may I help you?* Tap patient on shoulder or arm if you don't get a response.

2 Alert EMS.

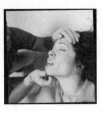

3 Put on barriers.

4 Practice opening airway using head tilt-chin lift (no head or spinal injuries suspected).

> Place one hand on patient's forehead and apply firm, backward pressure with your palm.

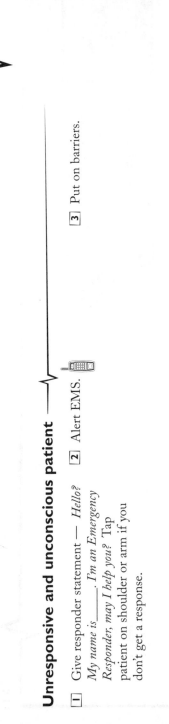

> Place the fingers of your other hand under the bony part of the lower jaw near the chin. Avoid pushing directly under the chin.

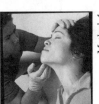

Method A

> Lift the jaw upward to bring the chin forward, tilting the entire head.

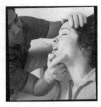

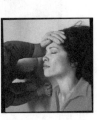

Method B

5 Practice opening airway using jaw thrust (head or spinal injuries suspected).

> Facing the top of the patient's head, rest your elbows on the surface on which the victim is lying.

> Grasp the angles of the patient's lower jaw and lift with both hands.

> If the lips are closed, you can retract the lower lip with your thumb.

> If rescue breathing is needed after looking, listening and feeling for breaths, close patient's nose by placing your cheek tightly against it or use a ventilation barrier that covers mouth and nose.

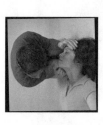

6 Look, listen and feel for breathing for up to 10 seconds.

> While holding the airway open, place your ear near patient's mouth – head turned toward patient's chest.

> Watch for chest movement.

> Listen for breathing sounds.

> Feel for air on your ear.

Unresponsive and unconscious patient (continued)

7 For breathing patient with possible spinal injury – immobilize head, neck and spine.

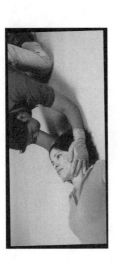

8 For breathing patient with no spinal injury – place in recovery position.

> Prepare to roll patient on side – lateral position. See photo for arm placement.

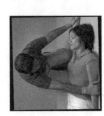

> Bring patient's top leg over and position on the ground in a bent position. Stabilize head and roll patient.

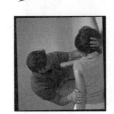

> Place patient's lower arm near or under the head for stabilization ensuring the airway remains open and unobstructed. See photo for final position.

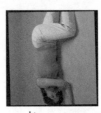

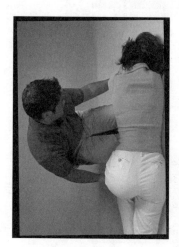

9 Look for serious bleeding.

10 Continue to monitor the ABCD'S and treat for shock.

Try It —∧— In your practice group, perform primary assessment on a responsive patient. One person is the guide, reading the steps, one is the patient, while the other is the Emergency Responder. Make sure everyone has the chance to act as the Emergency Responder. Then, practice primary assessment on an unresponsive, breathing patient, including use of the recovery position. Alter circumstances as directed by your instructor. Practice both the head tilt-chin lift and chin lift methods of opening an airway.

Primary Care Skill # 4
Rescue Breathing

Your Goal

Demonstrate how to perform adult rescue breathing that makes the chest rise using either the mouth-to-mouth or mouth-to-mask methods.

Key Points

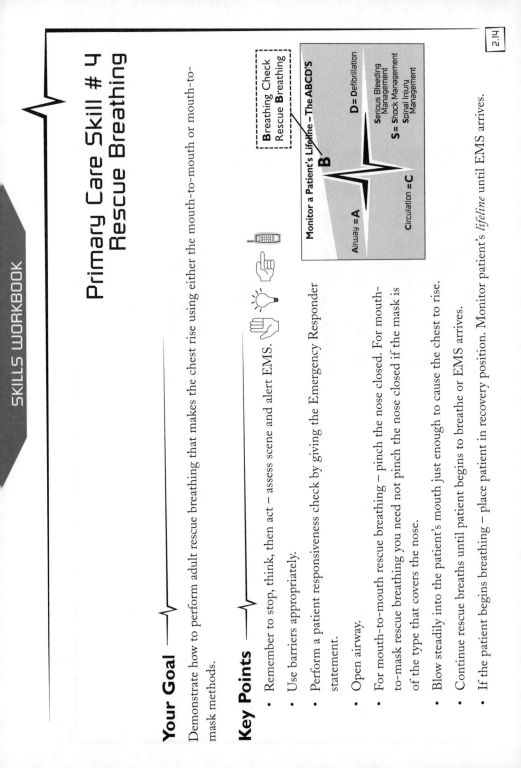

- Remember to stop, think, then act – assess scene and alert EMS.

- Use barriers appropriately.

- Perform a patient responsiveness check by giving the Emergency Responder statement.

- Open airway.

- For mouth-to-mouth rescue breathing – pinch the nose closed. For mouth-to-mask rescue breathing you need not pinch the nose closed if the mask is of the type that covers the nose.

- Blow steadily into the patient's mouth just enough to cause the chest to rise.

- Continue rescue breaths until patient begins to breathe or EMS arrives.

- If the patient begins breathing – place patient in recovery position. Monitor patient's *lifeline* until EMS arrives.

Monitor a Patient's Lifeline – The ABCD'S

Breathing Check
Rescue **B**reathing

B

Airway = **A**

Circulation = **C**

D = Defibrillation

Serious Bleeding Management
S = Shock Management
Spinal Injury Management

2.14

- It is important to note that adult patients who are not breathing more than likely have no heartbeat. You will probably have to perform CPR as well.

- If the patient shows no signs of circulation, begin chest compressions – This is practiced in Skill # 6 - One Rescuer, Adult CPR.

How It's Done

1 Give Emergency Responder statement. Assess scene and alert EMS.

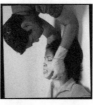

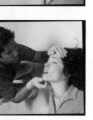

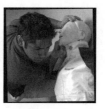

2 Airway open – head tilt-chin lift or chin lift method.

3 Breathing check – look, listen and feel for up to 10 seconds.

4 Position patient on back – remove obstructions from patient's mouth (loose dentures, chewing gum and other objects).

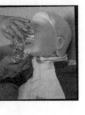
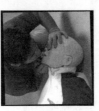
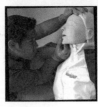

5 Position ventilation barrier for mouth-to-mouth or mouth-to-mask rescue breaths.

> If patient has an injury to the face or jaw, gently close the mouth to protect the injured site. While holding the jaw closed, place your mouth over the barrier covering the nose and give rescue breaths through the nose. Certain ventilation barriers are better for mouth-to-nose than others.

6 Rescue breathing – pinch nose closed and give two slow rescue breaths each lasting about two seconds.

7 More important than the breath lasting two seconds is the chest rising and falling with each breath. Maintain an open airway using either head tilt-chin lift or chin lift method.

> If you can't achieve two effective breaths, recheck airway for obstructions and proper position.

> Make up to five attempts to achieve effective breaths before assessing circulation.

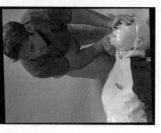

8. Check for signs of circulation for no more than 10 seconds – listening and feeling for breathing, plus scanning patient for any signs of movement.

9. If you determine the patient has a heartbeat, continue rescue breathing by giving one breath every five seconds. After one minute, again check for signs of circulation.

10. If patient begins to breathe on his own, continue to maintain an open airway. Place patient in the recovery position and continue to monitor the patient's *lifeline*.

Try It — In your practice group, perform rescue breathing on a mannequin using either the head tilt-chin lift or chin lift method to open the airway. One person is the guide, reading the steps, one watches, while the other is the Emergency Responder. Make sure everyone has the chance to act as the Emergency Responder. Alter circumstances as directed by your instructor.

Primary Care Skill # 5
One Rescuer, Adult CPR

Your Goals

· Conduct a circulation check to determine if a patient's heart is beating by noting patient movement, including swallowing or breathing.

· Perform One Rescuer, Adult CPR using proper body and hand placement at a rate of about 100 chest compressions per minute with a ratio of 15 compressions to two rescue breaths.

Key Points

· Remember to stop, think, then and act – assess scene and alert EMS.

· Use barriers appropriately.

· Perform a patient responsiveness check by giving the Emergency Responder statement.

· Open airway with head tilt-chin lift or chin lift method.

· Check for breathing – look, listen and feel for up to 10 seconds.

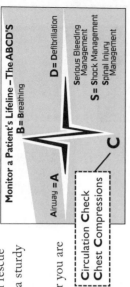

Monitor a Patient's Lifeline – The ABCD'S

Airway = **A**   **B** = Breathing

C

D = Defibrillation

Serious Bleeding Management
S = Shock Management
Spinal Injury Management

Circulation Check
Chest Compressions

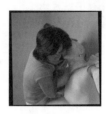

- If no breathing or circulation, begin One Rescuer, Adult CPR with rescue breathing. Remember that the patient must be on his back and on a sturdy surface.

- Continue CPR until the patient shows signs of life, EMS arrives or you are too exhausted to continue.

- Defibrillate when an Automated External Defibrillator (AED) is available and allowable (recommended skill) or EMS arrives.

How It's Done

1. Give Emergency Responder statement. Assess scene, alert EMS and make sure airway is open.

2. Conduct a breathing check and deliver two initial rescue breaths.

3. After initial rescue breaths, conduct a circulation check for no more than 10 seconds. To begin check:

   ✓ Place your ear near the patient's mouth – listen for breathing or coughing.

   ✓ Quickly scan patient for any movement. If no breathing, coughing or movement is detected, consider administering CPR.

Pulse Check

You might also try to feel for a carotid pulse. Locate patient's adam's apple with index and middle fingers, then slide fingers down into the groove of patient's neck on side closest to you. Remember, a circulation check should take no more than 10 total seconds. When in doubt about your abilities to find a carotid pulse, skip this check. Many people are unable to determine circulation, or the lack of a heartbeat, through a carotid pulse check – especially in older people.

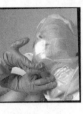

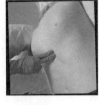

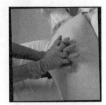

4 If no circulation is detected, locate the compression site by one of two techniques. Technique one:

> Place your fingers on the lower margin of the patient's rib cage on the side nearer you.

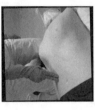

> Slide your fingers up the rib cage to the notch where the ribs meet the lower breastbone (sternum) in the center of the lower part of the chest.

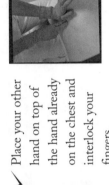

> Place the heel of one hand on the lower half of the breastbone next to two fingers.

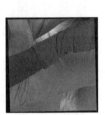

> Place your other hand on top of the hand already on the chest and interlock your fingers.

2.20

5 Use technique two if you forget technique one or have trouble with technique one:

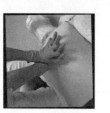

> Place the heel of one hand in the center of the chest between the nipples.

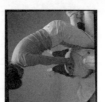

> Place your other hand on top of the hand already on the chest and interlock your fingers.

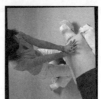

6 Position your shoulders directly over your hands – arms straight with elbows locked. Keep the force of the compression straight down – avoid pushing on the rib cage or the lower tip of the breast bone.

7 Maintaining this position, press down on sternum with enough force to depress it between 4–5 centimetres/1.5–2 inches.

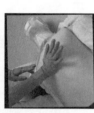

8 Release the pressure and repeat for 15 compressions at a rate of 100 compressions per minute. Each time you compress the chest, count One and Two and Three and Four... etc. More important than putting the word "and" between the numeric counting is keeping the proper compression rate.

9 After 15 compressions, open patient's airway and administer two rescue breaths.

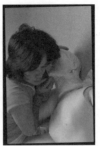

10 Return your hands to the proper position and give 15 additional compressions followed by two rescue breaths.

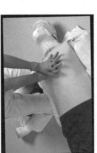

11 After approximately one minute (about four cycles of two breaths to 15 compressions), check for signs of circulation. If still absent, continue CPR.

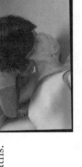

Try It 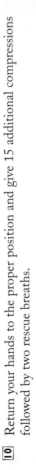 In your practice group perform One Rescuer, Adult CPR on a mannequin. One person is the guide, reading the steps, one watches, while the other is the Emergency Responder. Each Emergency Responder should:

✓ First, practice the steps slowly to make sure his hand, arm and body position is appropriate.

✓ Next, practice the steps again in real time.

Make sure everyone has the chance to act as the Emergency Responder. Alter circumstances as directed by your instructor.

Primary Care Skill # 6
Serious Bleeding Management

Your Goal

Demonstrate how to use direct pressure, a pressure bandage and a pressure point to manage a serious bleeding wound.

Key Points

- Remember to stop, think, then act – assess scene and alert EMS.

- Use barriers appropriately. For serious bleeding, appropriate barriers include gloves, eye shield, personal face mask and ventilation shield.

- Perform a patient responsiveness check by giving the Emergency Responder statement.

- Perform a primary assessment – remember bleeding must be severe to be life threatening.

- Keep in mind that direct pressure is the first and most successful method for serious bleeding management.

- Using a pressure bandage is the next step to control bleeding. A pressure bandage is anything that places constant direct pressure on a wound.

- Elevate the bleeding area if possible.

- For arterial bleeding it may be necessary to use a pressure point in addition to direct pressure and a pressure bandage to decrease blood flow. A pressure point is an area of the body where an artery lies next to a bone.

How It's Done

Direct Pressure

1. Give Emergency Responder statement. Assess scene, alert EMS and make sure airway is open.

2. Put on barriers.

3. Place a clean cloth or a sterile dressing over wound and apply pressure.

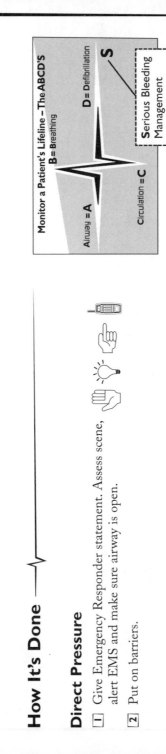

4. Release pressure periodically to determine if bleeding has slowed or stopped.

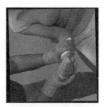

5. Elevate wound to assist in the control of bleeding.

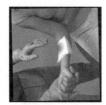

Monitor a Patient's Lifeline — The ABCD'S

Airway = **A**

B = Breathing

Circulation = **C**

D = Defibrillation

S

Serious Bleeding Management

Pressure Bandage

1 While applying direct pressure on wound, place a pressure bandage over the sterile dressing.

2 If bandage becomes blood-soaked, place another clean cloth or dressing on top and bandage in place.

3 Continue to apply direct pressure to wound and elevate to assist in bleeding control.

4 Don't remove blood-soaked bandages because blood clots in the dressing help control bleeding. Add bandages as necessary.

5 Bandage rather tightly – avoiding total restriction of blood flow (no discoloring of fingers or toes).

Pressure Point

1 If direct pressure is not adequate for arterial bleeding, determine which body pressure point will slow the flow of blood to the wound – leg or arm.

2. While maintaining direct pressure on wound, apply pressure with your fingers, thumb, or the heel of your other hand to the appropriate pressure point.

> Press artery against the bone and observe if bleeding slows.

> If not, reposition hand and try again.

> Hold pressure point long enough to allow clotting to occur.

> To check, slowly release pressure to see if strong flow returns.

> Continue direct pressure and pressure point use until EMS arrives.

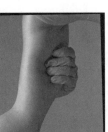

Brachial Artery pressure point.

Try It — In your practice group begin by performing a primary assessment and attend to an imaginary serious bleeding wound on a patient's arm. Progress from direct pressure to a pressure bandage to applying a pressure point on the brachial artery (on the arm; see photo). Patient should monitor their wrist pulse to feel effectiveness of pressure point. One person is the guide, reading the steps, one acts as a patient with a wound, while the other is the Emergency Responder.

Make sure everyone has the chance to act as the Emergency Responder. Alter circumstances as directed by your instructor.

Primary Care Skill # 7
Shock Management

Your Goal

Demonstrate how to manage shock by conducting a primary assessment, protecting the patient and stabilizing the head.

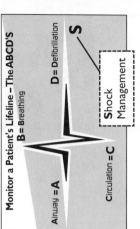

Monitor a Patient's Lifeline – The ABCD'S

Airway = A

B = Breathing

D = Defibrillation

Circulation = C

S

Shock Management

Key Points

- Remember to stop, think and act – assess scene and alert EMS.

- Use barriers appropriately.

- Perform a patient responsiveness check by giving the responder statement.

- Perform a primary assessment. Monitor a patient's *lifeline*.

- Shock results when an injury or illness makes it difficult for the body's cardiovascular system to provide adequate amounts of oxygenated blood to vital organs.

- Always treat an injured or ill patient for shock even if signs and symptoms are absent.

- For a responsive patient, let the patient determine what position is most comfortable – sitting, lying down, etc.

How It's Done

1 Treat an injured, unresponsive or unconscious patient in the position found. Do not move.

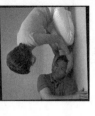

2 Hold the patient's head to keep the neck from moving.

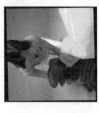

3 Maintain patient's body temperature based on local climate. This may mean covering the patient with a blanket or exposure protection from the sun.

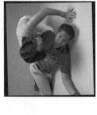

4 If there are no spinal injuries or leg fractures suspected, elevate the legs 15-30 centimetres/6-12 inches to allow blood to return to the heart.

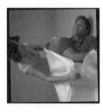

Try It

In your practice group begin by performing a primary assessment and manage shock for an unconscious patient laying on the floor. Cover with a blanket or shade the patient to provide a normal temperature. Elevate the patient's legs 15-30 centimetres/6-12 inches. One person is the guide, reading the steps, one acts as a patient with shock, while the other is the Emergency Responder. Be resourceful, use items in the room to shade or cover patient and elevate legs.

Make sure everyone has the chance to act as the Emergency Responder. Alter circumstances as directed by your instructor.

Primary Care Skill # 8
Spinal Injury Management

Your Goal

Demonstrate how to manage a suspected spinal injury by conducting a primary assessment, protecting the patient and stabilizing the head.

Key Points

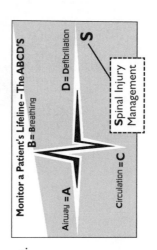

- Remember to stop, think and act – assess scene and alert EMS.

- Use barriers appropriately.

- Perform a patient responsiveness check by giving the responder statement.

- Suspect a spinal injury for any incident involving a fall, severe blow, crash or other strong impact.

- If possible, perform primary assessment in the position the patient is found. Do not move patient unless safety is in question. Monitor the patient's *lifeline*.

How It's Done

For a conscious and responsive patient

1. Stabilize head by placing a hand on each side to prevent movement.

2. Instruct patient to remain still and not move his head or neck while waiting for EMS to arrive.

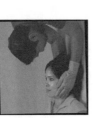

For an unconscious and unresponsive patient

1. To open airway, assess breathing, administer rescue breaths or CPR, patient must be on his back.

> If patient is already on his back, use the jaw thrust method to open patient's airway. Do not tilt head back or turn it from side to side.

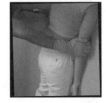

> If patient is not on his back, use the log roll to reposition patient.

To perform a log roll by yourself:

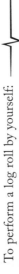

> Kneel at the patient's side. Leave enough room so that patient will not roll into your lap.

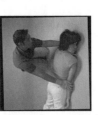

> Gently straighten patient's legs. Straighten arms against side of patient.

> Cradle patient's head and neck from behind with one of your hands.

✓ Place your other hand on patient's elbow – on the patient's arm that is furthest away from you.

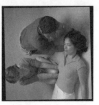

✓ Roll patient as carefully as possible. Roll patient as a unit toward you, onto his side, then onto his back.

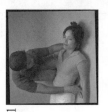

If help is available, perform a two-person log roll:

✓ One Emergency Responder stabilizes patient's head, one rolls patient. Patient's head is stabilized with both hands to keep it from moving.

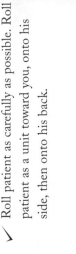

✓ Emergency Responder rolling patient, does so with both hands on patient's arm above and below elbow.

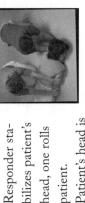

✓ Both responders roll patient as one unit onto patient's back.

Try It ⚡ In your practice group begin by performing a primary assessment on a responsive patient with a suspected spinal injury. Next, practice a log roll and primary assessment on an unconscious and unresponsive patient with a suspected spinal injury who is positioned face down.

If practical, practice both two-person and one-person log rolls. One person is the guide, reading the steps, one acts as a patient with a spinal injury, while the other is the Emergency Responder.

Make sure everyone has the chance to act as the Emergency Responder. Alter circumstances as directed by your instructor.

Recommended Primary Care Skill
Automated External Defibrillator

Your Goal

Demonstrate how to:

- Use an Automated External Defibrillator (AED) on a mannequin according to the machine manufacturer's guidelines.

- Place AED pads on a patient with no signs of circulation.

- Assist a patient who has been successfully defibrillated with an AED.

Key Points

- An AED is a sophisticated, microprocessor-based device that incorporates a heart rhythm analysis and a shock-advisory system.

- In some regions, AED use by laypersons may be restricted.

- Remember to stop, think and act – assess scene and alert EMS.

- Protect yourself and patient from disease transmission by using barriers.

- Perform a patient responsiveness check by giving the responder statement and then, if unresponsive, tapping the shoulder or arm.

- Perform a primary assessment including checking for signs of circulation.

- Begin CPR and continue until AED is available. **If AED is available immediately, begin with its use as soon as possible.**

- If needed, prepare chest by wiping off water or shaving hair where pads are placed.

- Never place AED pads over pacemakers – place them two cm/one inch away.

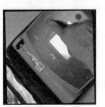

Monitor a Patient's Lifeline – The ABCD'S

Airway = **A**

B = Breathing

Defibrillation - By EMS or AED

D

Circulation = **C**

Serious Bleeding Management
S = Shock Management
Spinal Injury Management

How It's Done

1 Treat patient's *lifeline.* Continue to perform CPR until AED arrives.

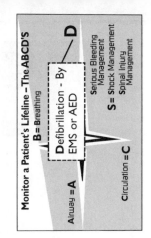

2 Stop CPR and position AED close to the patient's ear – left side of patient is preferable for easy access to AED controls and easy pad placement.

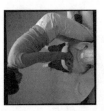

3 Turn AED power ON – follow device prompts.

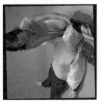

4 Remove defibrillator pads from packaging – peel away any protective plastic backing from the pads.

5 As directed by manufacturer, place defibrillator pads on patient's bare chest, adhesive side down (note placement illustrations on pad packaging or pads). Typically:

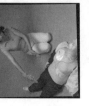

> One pad goes on the upper-right side of chest, below the collarbone, next to breastbone.

> One pad goes on lower-left side of the chest, below nipple line.

6 Plug in AED if needed or prompted. AED analyzes patient's heart rhythm. (Some AEDs require you push an *Analyze* button.)

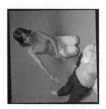

7 Clear rescuers and bystanders from the patient making sure no one is touching the patient. Also, make sure no equipment is touching the patient. Say, *I'm clear, you are clear, everybody clear.*

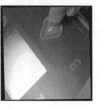

8 If defibrillation is required, the AED prompt will inform you to shock patient.

9 Loudly announce, *Stand Clear* or *Clear.* Do not touch the patient. Scan the patient to make sure no one is touching the patient.

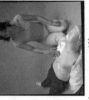

10 Push button and administer shock to the patient. AED will again analyze patient. Do not reinitiate CPR after initial shock, touch the patient or interfere with the analysis of the AED.

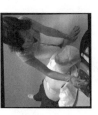

11 Repeat shocks as prompted by the AED.

12 Perform circulation check and shock patient as prompted by AED.

13 Perform CPR for one minute after each group of three shocks with AED still attached.

14 If signs of circulation return and AED indicates no further shock needed:

✓ Place patient in recovery position – monitor breathing and signs of circulation.

✓ Leave AED attached to patient.

✓ Continue to follow AED prompts.

15 If no shock is indicated by AED but patient shows no signs of circulation:

✓ Start CPR with AED still attached.

✓ After one minute of CPR, analyze again with AED.

Try It

In your practice group, place AED pads on a mannequin and proceed through the Analyze and Shock steps. One person is the guide, reading the steps, one watches, while the other is the Emergency Responder. Each Emergency Responder should:

✓ Practice AED pad placement.

✓ Practice on an AED Trainer or simulate the steps for analyzing and shocking a patient (mannequin).

Make sure everyone has the chance to act as the Emergency Responder. Alter circumstances as directed by your instructor.

Americas Version

Recommended Primary Care Skill
Conscious/Unconscious Choking Adult

Your Goal

Demonstrate how to assist a conscious choking patient with a partial or complete airway obstruction.

Key Points

- Remember to stop, think, then act – assess scene and alert EMS.

- If the patient is coughing, wheezing or can speak, observe until the patient expels the obstruction. Reassure and encourage the patient to keep coughing to expel the foreign material.

- Remember that a conscious adult must give consent before you do anything. A head nod is sufficient.

- Perform chest thrusts on pregnant or obese individuals rather than abdominal thrusts.

- Patients who receive the treatment for conscious choking (abdominal and chest thrusts), should be medically evaluated to rule out any life threatening complications.

Special Note

Procedures for handling choking – both when an adult is conscious or becomes unconscious – vary internationally. Your instructor will advise you on protocols appropriate for your area. Three variations are listed here – Americas, Asia Pacific and Europe.

Monitor a Patient's Lifeline – The ABCD'S

Airway = **A**

B = Breathing

Circulation = **C**

D = Defibrillation

Serious Bleeding Management

S = Shock Management
Spinal Injury Management

How It's Done

1 Ask, *Are you choking?*

2 If patient is not coughing and can't speak, give responder statement. *Hello? My name is _____. I'm an Emergency Responder, may I help you?*

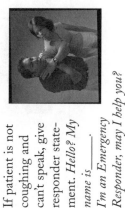

3 When permission is granted, use the local protocol for assisting a conscious choking adult.

Conscious Choking Abdominal Thrusts (Heimlich Maneuver)

1 Stand behind patient and place arms around waist.

2 Locate patient's navel — the thrust site is two finger widths above it.

3 Make a fist and place thumb side on the thrust site.

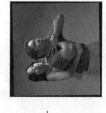

4 Place other hand over the outside of fist.

5 Bend arms and elbows outward to avoid squeezing ribcage.

6 Perform quick inward and upward thrusts until object is expelled or patient loses consciousness.

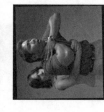

NOTE: DO NOT PERFORM THE THRUSTS FULL FORCE IN CLASS. Practice performing the thrusts lightly.

Conscious Choking Chest Thrusts (also for pregnant or obese individuals)

1 Stand behind patient and place arms around body, under arm pits.

2 Follow lowest rib upward until you reach the point where ribs meet in the center.

3 Feel notch on the lower half of breast bone – sternum – place your middle and index finger on the notch.

4 Make a fist and place thumb side on the thrust site above notch.

5 Place other hand over the outside of the fist.

6 At this point you would perform quick inward thrusts until object is expelled or patient loses consciousness.

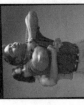

7 Avoid putting pressure on the rib cage. Use this technique for pregnant or obese individuals.

NOTE: DO NOT PERFORM THE THRUSTS FULL FORCE IN CLASS. Practice performing the thrusts lightly.

Unconscious (caused by choking) Patient

1 Open airway with head tilt, remove any visible obstruction from mouth then continue with chin lift.

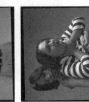

2 Perform breathing check.

3 Attempt two effective rescue breaths.

4 Give two rescue breaths within five attempts, check for signs of circulation. Start chest compressions and/or rescue breathing as appropriate.

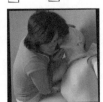

5 If can't achieve two rescue breaths, start chest compressions immediately to relieve obstruction. Do not check for signs of circulation. After 15 compressions, check mouth for visible obstruction and attempt two rescue breaths. Continue at 15:2 compressions to rescue breaths.

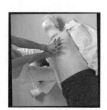

6 If you achieve rescue breaths at any time, check for signs of circulation and continue chest compressions and/or rescue breathing as appropriate.

Try It ⎯⌁⎯ In your practice group, perform the steps to assist a conscious choking patient. One person is the guide, reading the steps, one is the patient, while the other is the Emergency Responder. Make sure everyone has the chance to act as the Emergency Responder. *Remember – Do not actually perform thrusts or blows for practice.* Next, discuss and/or perform the steps for assisting a patient who has become unconscious from a choking incident – back blows and/or lateral chest thrusts or CPR. Your instructor will direct you. Alter circumstances as directed by your instructor.

Europe Version

Primary Care Skill #9
Conscious/Unconscious Choking Adult

Your Goal

Demonstrate how to assist a conscious choking patient with a partial or complete airway obstruction.

Key Points

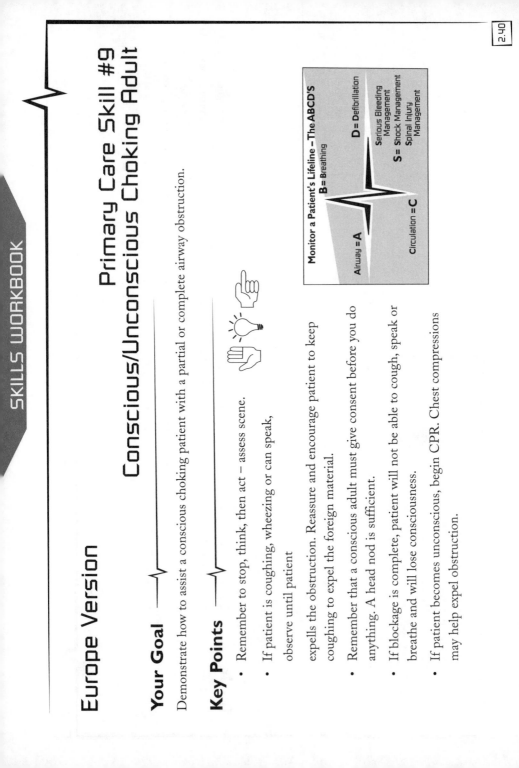

- Remember to stop, think, then act – assess scene.

- If patient is coughing, wheezing or can speak, observe until patient

  expels the obstruction. Reassure and encourage patient to keep coughing to expel the foreign material.

- Remember that a conscious adult must give consent before you do anything. A head nod is sufficient.

- If blockage is complete, patient will not be able to cough, speak or breathe and will lose consciousness.

- If patient becomes unconscious, begin CPR. Chest compressions may help expel obstruction.

Monitor a Patient's Lifeline – The ABCD'S

Airway = **A**

B = Breathing

Circulation = **C**

D = Defibrillation

Serious Bleeding Management

S = Shock Management

Spinal Injury Management

- Perform chest thrusts rather than abdominal thrusts on pregnant or obese individuals.
- Patients who receive treatment for conscious choking (abdominal and chest thrusts), should be medically evaluated to rule out any life-threatening complications.

How It's Done

[1] Encourage patient to continue coughing. Reassure.

[2] If patient is not coughing and can't speak, give Emergency Responder statement. *Hello? My name is_____. I'm an Emergency Responder, may I help you?*

Conscious Choking Back Blows

[3] Perform back blows as follows:

> Remove any obvious obstructions from the mouth.

> Stand to the side and slightly behind the patient.

> Supporting the chest with one hand, lean the patient well forwards.

> Give up to five sharp blows between shoulder blades with heel of hand.

> Stop if obstruction clears.

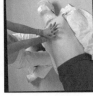

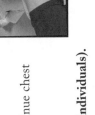

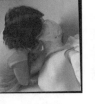

Unconscious (caused by choking) Patient

1. Open airway with head tilt, remove any visible obstruction from mouth then continue with chin lift.

2. Perform breathing check.

3. Attempt two effective rescue breaths.

4. Give two rescue breaths within five attempts, check for signs of circulation. Start chest compressions and/or rescue breathing as appropriate.

5. If can't achieve two rescue breaths, start chest compressions immediately to relieve obstruction. Do not check for signs of circulation. After 15 compressions, check mouth for visible obstruction and attempt two rescue breaths. Continue at 15:2 compressions to rescue breaths.

6. If you achieve rescue preaths at any time, check for signs of circulation and continue chest compressions and/or rescue breathing as appropriate.

Conscious Choking Chest Thrusts (for use on pregnant or obese individuals).

1. Replaces abdominal thrusts in sequence for conscious choking adults.

2. Stand behind patient and place arms around body, under arpits.

3. Follow lowest rib upward until the point where ribs meet in the centre.

4. Feel notch on lower half of breastbond (sternum), then place middle and index finger on notch.

5. Make a fist and place thumb side on the thrust site above notch.

6. Place other hand over outside of fist.

7. Perform up to five quick inward and upward thrusts.

8. Avoid putting pressure on rib cage.

Try It — In your practise group, perform the steps to assist a conscious choking patient. One person is the guide, reading the steps, one is the patient, while the other is the Emergency Responder. Make sure everyone has the chance to act as the Emergency Responder. *Remember – Do not actually perform thrusts or blows for practise.* Next, discuss and/or perform the steps for assisting a patient who has become unconscious from a choking incident – back blows and/or lateral chest thrusts or CPR. Your instructor will direct you. Alter circumstances as directed by your instructor.

Asia Pacific Version

Primary Care Skill #14
Conscious/Unconscious Choking Adult

Your Goal

Demonstrate how to assist a conscious choking adult patient with a partial airway obstruction and an unconscious choking patient with a total airway obstruction.

Key Points

- Remember to stop, think, then act – assess scene and alert EMS.

- If the patient is coughing, wheezing or can speak, observe until he expels the obstruction. Reassure and encourage the patient to keep coughing and to try to expel the foreign material. If the partial obstruction persists for more than a few minutes, stay with the patient and send others to alert EMS.

- Remember that a conscious adult must give consent before you do anything. A head nod is sufficient.

- Patients who receive treatment for choking (back blows or chest and abdominal thrusts), should be medically evaluated to rule out any life-threatening complications.

Monitor a Patient's Lifeline – The **ABCD'S**

Airway = **A**

B = Breathing

Circulation = **C**

D = Defibrillation

Serious Bleeding Management

S = Shock Management

Spinal Injury Management

How It's Done

1 Ask, *Are you choking?*

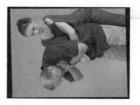

2 If patient is coughing and wheezing, but can't speak, give Emergency Responder statement. *Hello? My name is_____. I'm an Emergency Responder, may I help you?*

3 When permission is granted, continue to reassure and encourage the patient to relax and to keep coughing to try and expel the foreign material. Have patient breathe deeply.

Conscious Choking Back Blows for Total Blockage

1 If patient is unsuccessful at coughing up the total obstruction:

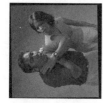

✓ Bend patient forward.

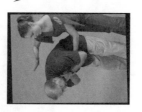

✓ Deliver five sharp back blows between shoulder blades using heel of hand.

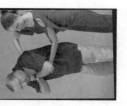

✓ If patient is still choking, proceed to abdominal thrusts (New Zealand only).

NOTE: DO NOT PERFORM BACK BLOWS FULL FORCE IN CLASS. Practise performing back blows lightly.

Conscious Choking Abdominal Thrusts (New Zealand)

1 Stand behind patient and place arms around waist.

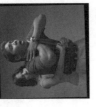

2 Locate patient's navel – the thrust site is two finger widths above it.

3 Make a fist and place thumb side on the thrust site.

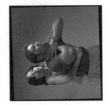

4 Place other hand over the outside of fist.

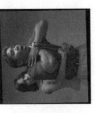

5 Bend arms and elbows outward to avoid squeezing ribcage.

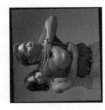

6 Perform quick inward and upward thrusts until object is expelled or patient loses consciousness. If the patient loses consciousness, call EMS and begin standard CPR. Check the airway for an obstruction prior to rescue breathing.

NOTE: DO NOT PERFORM THE THRUSTS FULL FORCE IN CLASS. Practice performing the thrusts lightly.

Unconscious Patient Back Blows for Total Blockage (Australia) —√—

1 If the patient is already unconscious or becomes unconscious, begin back blows.

√ Turn patient on side – attempt to clear and open airway.

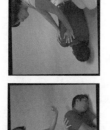

√ Check for signs of breathing. No breathing – give up to four sharp back blows between the shoulder blades using heel of hand.

√ Re-check for signs of breathing. If none, proceed to lateral chest thrusts.

NOTE: DO NOT PERFORM BACK BLOWS FULL FORCE IN CLASS. Practise performing back blows lightly.

Unconscious Patient Lateral Chest Thrusts (Australia) —√—

1 Keep patient on side.

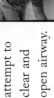

2 Place one hand against lower fold of patient's armpit.

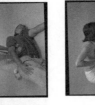

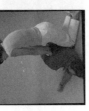

3 Place other hand beside the first and give up to four quick, downward thrusts keeping your hands on the chest throughout. Avoid applying pressure below the ribcage.

4 Clear and open patient's airway – re-check for signs of breathing. Repeat thrusts and breathing checks if obstruction persists.

5 Alert EMS if back blows and lateral thrusts are unsuccessful in removing obstruction.

NOTE: DO NOT PERFORM THRUSTS FULL FORCE IN CLASS. Practise performing the thrusts lightly.

Try It ⎯∿⎯ In your practise group, perform the steps to assist a conscious and *unconscious* choking patient. One person is the guide, reading the steps, one is the patient, while the other is the Emergency Responder. Make sure everyone has the chance to act as the Emergency Responder. Remember – Do not actually perform blows or thrusts for practise. Your instructor will direct you. Alter circumstances as directed by your instructor.

Recommended Primary Care Skill
Emergency Oxygen Use

Your Goal

Demonstrate how to administer emergency oxygen to a patient with a serious or life threatening illness or injury.

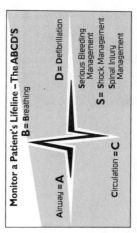

Monitor a Patient's Lifeline – The ABCD'S

Airway = A

B = Breathing

Circulation = C

D = Defibrillation

Serious Bleeding Management

S = Shock Management
Spinal Injury Management

Key Points

- Remember to stop, think, then act – assess scene and alert EMS.

- Use barriers appropriately.

- Perform a patient responsiveness check by giving the responder statement.

- Perform a primary assessment. Monitor the patient's *lifeline*.

- Become familiar with the emergency oxygen units that you may need to use before you need to use them – at home, work, school, etc.

- Use emergency oxygen in a ventilated area away from any source of flame or heat.

- Handle oxygen cylinder carefully because contents are under high pressure. Avoid dropping cylinder or exposing it to heat.

- In some regions, oxygen use is restricted.

How It's Done

1. Follow system instructions to set up oxygen unit.

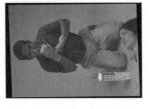

2. Always turn valve on slowly and test that oxygen is flowing to mask.

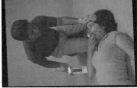

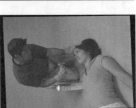

3. For a responsive patient, ask if you may provide oxygen and place mask over the patient's mouth and nose. Say, *This is oxygen, may I help you?* Responder takes first breath from mask, but does not exhale.

✓ If the patient agrees, have the patient hold the mask in place and tell the patient to breathe normally.

✓ If the patient can't hold the mask, use the strap to keep it in place.

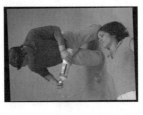

4 For a nonresponsive, breathing patient, place mask on patient's nose and mouth and secure with strap.

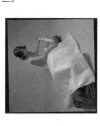

5 For an unconscious, nonbreathing patient, use a mask that allows you to supply rescue breaths while oxygen flows into mask.

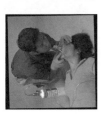

6 Monitor oxygen unit pressure gauge to avoid emptying it while the mask is still on the patient.

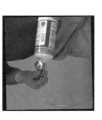

Try It — In your practice group, set up an oxygen unit following your instructor's directions. Next, perform a primary assessment on a responsive patient. One person is the guide, reading the steps, one is the patient, while the other is the Emergency Responder. Offer patient emergency oxygen following your instructor's directions.

Make sure everyone has the chance to act as the Emergency Responder. Alter circumstances as directed by your instructor.

Secondary Care (First Aid)

Secondary Care Skill # 1
Injury Assessment

Your Goal

Demonstrate how to conduct a head-to-toe injury assessment on a patient and note injuries to report to Emergency Medical Service (EMS) personnel.

Key Points

- Use this skill to determine what first aid may be needed in the event of any injury – especially when Emergency Medical Service is either delayed or unavailable.

- Remember to stop, think, then act – assess scene and alert EMS if necessary.

- Use barriers appropriately.

- Perform a patient responsiveness check by giving the responder statement.

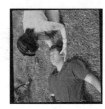

Monitor a Patient's Lifeline – The ABCD'S

Airway = **A**

B = Breathing

D = Defibrillation
Serious Bleeding
Management

S = Shock Management
Spinal Injury
Management

Circulation = **C**

- Perform a primary assessment and monitor and treat the patient's *lifeline* if needed.

- Only perform injury assessments on conscious, responsive patients.

- When possible, perform the assessment in the position the patient is found.

- If wound dressings are in place, do not remove during the assessment.

- Look for wounds, bleeding, discolorations or deformities.

- Listen for unusual breathing sounds.

- Feel for swelling or hardness, tissue softness, unusual masses, joint tenderness, deformities and changes in body temperature. Make mental notes of the assessment and report findings to EMS personnel.

- Avoid giving injured patient anything to eat or drink as he may need surgery.

How It's Done

1 Deliver responder statement, asking permission to assist. Give a brief explanation of what you'll be doing during the assessment. Put on gloves.

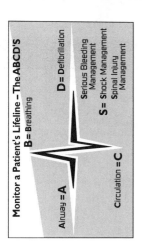

2 Stabilize patient's head and instruct patient to answer verbally. Do not allow patient to move or nod head.

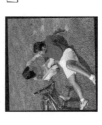

3 Immediately stop assessment if patient complains of head, neck or back pain. Continue to stabilize head and neck – ending assessment and waiting for EMS to arrive. Do not move.

4 Start assessment at head and work your way down body to toes.

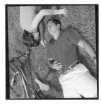
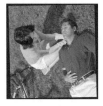

5 Feel for deformities on patient's face by gently running your fingers over forehead, cheeks and chin.

6 Check ears and nose for blood or fluid. If present, suspect head injury and stop further assessment.

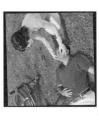
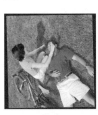

7 Place a finger in front of patient's eyes. Without moving the head, have patient follow your finger with his eyes. Check eyes for smooth tracking. Eyes should move together. If possible, check pupil size and reaction to light.

8 Feel skull and neck for abnormalities. If patient complains of pain, stop assessment.

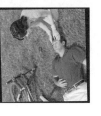

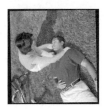

9 If you can reach the shoulder blades, slide or place one hand over each shoulder blade and gently push inwards.

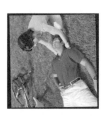

11 Run two fingers over the collarbones from shoulders to center.

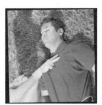

13 Inspect chest for deformity. Place a hand, palm in, on each side of patient's ribcage and gently push inward.

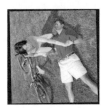

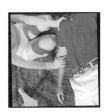

10 Move hands outward to shoulders and press gently inward with palm.

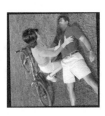

12 Place one hand on shoulder to stabilize arm. Gently slide other hand down the upper arm, elbow and wrist. Repeat on other arm. Ask patient to wiggle fingers on both hands and squeeze your hands.

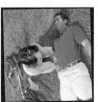

14 Gently put your hands under patient to feel the spinal column. Cover as much area as possible without moving patient. Gently touch along the patient's spine, feeling for abnormalities.

15 Using one hand, gently push on patient's abdomen. Apply gentle pressure to right and left side of abdomen, and above and below navel.

16 Move hands over hip bones, palms inward, and gently push in on hips.

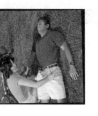

17 Starting at the thigh, slide hand down the upper leg, knee, lower leg and ankle. Ask patient to wiggle toes and press sole of the foot against your hand. Repeat on other leg.

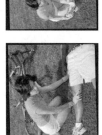

18 Note areas of pain or abnormality for report to EMS personnel. Continue to monitor and treat patient's *lifeline.*

Try It

In your practice group, perform a primary assessment on a responsive patient. Next, begin your Injury Assessment. In this situation, EMS is either delayed or unavailable.

One person is the guide, reading the steps, one is the patient, while the other is the Emergency Responder. Each patient should *think* of an imaginary injury. Do not share this imaginary injury with the Emergency Responder. As the Emergency Responder performs his Injury Assessment, *act out* the injury.

Make sure everyone has the chance to act as the Emergency Responder. Alter circumstances as directed by your instructor.

Secondary Care Skill # 2
Illness Assessment

Your Goal

Demonstrate how to conduct an illness assessment by:

- Asking how a patient feels and obtaining information about a patient's medical history.
- Checking a patient's respirations, pulse rate, temperature, skin moisture and color.
- Reporting findings to Emergency Medical Service (EMS) personnel.

Key Points

- Use this skill to gather information and determine what first aid may be needed in the event of any illness – especially when Emergency Medical Service is either delayed or unavailable.

- Stop, think, then act – assess scene and alert EMS if necessary.

- Protect yourself and patient from disease transmission by using gloves and barriers.

- Perform a patient responsiveness check by giving the responder statement.

- Perform a primary assessment and monitor and treat the patient's *lifeline* if needed.

- Only perform illness assessments on conscious, responsive patients.

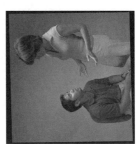

Monitor a Patient's Lifeline – The ABCD'S

Airway = **A**

B = Breathing

Circulation = **C**

D = Defibrillation

S = Serious Bleeding Management
Shock Management
Spinal Injury Management

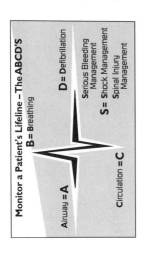

- When giving information to EMS personnel, avoid using the word *normal*. Provide measured rates per minute and descriptive terminology.

- Use the mnemonic SAMPLE to remember how to conduct an illness assessment. SAMPLE stands for **S**igns and **S**ymptoms, **A**llergies, **M**edications, **P**reexisting medical history, **L**ast meal and **E**vents.

- Signs are something you *see* is wrong with a patient. Symptoms are something the patient *tells* you is wrong.

- To help guide your assessment, remember that:

  › The average breathing rate for adults is between 12 and 20 breaths per minute. A patient who takes less than eight breaths per minute, or more than 24 breaths per minute, probably needs immediate medical care.

  › The average pulse rate for adults is between 60-80 beats per minute.

  › Average skin temperature is warm and skin should feel dry to the touch.

  › Noticeable skin color changes may indicate heart, lung or circulation problems.

  › By conducting an illness assessment on a healthy person in class, you will be able to recognize differences later when you assist an unhealthy person.

How It's Done

1. Find a paper and a pen/pencil to record illness assessment information. Use the Illness Assessment Record Sheet at the end of the *Reference* section.

2. If possible, have someone else record information.

3. Put on gloves when needed.

SAMPLE – Signs and Symptoms

1. Ask how patient is feeling and what occurred immediately before the onset of illness. Questions may include:

  - How do you feel now?

  - What were you doing when you began to feel ill?

  - When did the first symptoms occur?

  - Where were you when the first symptoms occurred?

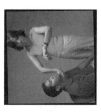

Finding Pulse Rate

2. To find pulse rate using the carotid artery:

  - Locate the patient's Adam's apple with the index and middle fingers of one hand.

  - Slide the fingers down into the groove of the neck on the side closest to you.

  - If you can't find the pulse on the side closest to you, move to the opposite side.

⟩ Never try to feel the carotid pulse on both sides at the same time.

⟩ Count the number of beats in 30 seconds and multiply by two to determine the heartbeats per minute.

3 To find pulse rate using the radial artery:

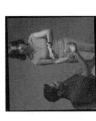

⟩ Locate artery on patient's wrist, thumb side of hand.

⟩ Slide two or three fingers into the groove of the wrist immediately below the hand on the thumb side.

⟩ Do not use your thumb when taking a radial pulse.

⟩ Count the number of beats in 30 seconds and multiply by two to determine the heartbeats per minute.

4 Determine whether the pulse may be described as rapid, strong or weak.

Checking Respiration

5 Look for signs and symptoms of respiratory distress, including:

⟩ Wheezing, gurgling or high-pitched noises when the patient breathes.

⟩ Patient complains of shortness of breath or feeling dizzy or lightheaded.

⟩ Patient complains of pain in the chest and numbness or tingling in arms or legs.

6. To count the number of times a patient breathes, use one of two methods:

✓ First Method: Simply watch patient's chest rise and fall and count the respirations.

✓ Second Method: If you cannot see the patient's chest rise and fall, place hand on the patient's abdomen. This position allows you to mask your efforts to obtain a count of the patient's respirations. Patients often alter their breathing rate if they become aware their breaths are being counted.

✓ For both methods, count patient's respirations for 30 seconds and multiply by two to determine respiratory rate.

7. Determine whether respirations may be described as fast, slow, labored, wheezing or gasping.

Checking temperature and moisture

8. Feel patient's forehead or cheek with the back of your hand. Compare with your own temperature using your other hand on your forehead. Verify if the patient has perhaps been doing physical exercise.

9. Determine whether the skin is warm, hot, cool, moist, clammy, etc.

Determining Color

10. Look for apparent skin color changes that may be described as extremely pale, ashen (grey), red, blue, yellowish or black-and-blue blotches.

11. If the patient has dark skin, check for color changes on the nailbeds, lips, gums, tongue, palms, whites of the eyes and ear lobes.

SAMPLE – Allergies

1. Ask if patient is allergic to anything – food, drugs, airborne matter, etc.

2. Ask if patient my have ingested or taken anything the patient is allergic to.

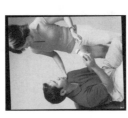

SAMPLE – Medications

1. Ask if patient takes medication for a medical condition. Questions may include:

    - Do you take medication?

    - If yes, what type of medication do you take?

    - Did you take medication today?

    - How much medication did you take and when?

2. If possible, collect all medication to give to EMS personnel and/or get name of the doctor who prescribed the medication.

SAMPLE – Preexisting Medical Conditions

1. Ask if patient has a preexisting medical condition (e.g., heart condition, diabetes, asthma, epilepsy, etc.)

SAMPLE – Last Meal

☐ Ask when patient last had a meal and what patient ate. Ask if he has consumed any alcohol or recreational drugs.

SAMPLE – Events

☐ Ask patient about or note events leading up to illness.

Try It — In your practice group, perform a primary assessment on a responsive patient. Next, begin your Illness Assessment. In this situation, EMS is either delayed or unavailable.

One person is the guide, reading the steps, one is the patient, while the other is the Emergency Responder conducting the illness assessment. By conducting an illness assessment on a healthy person in class, you will be able to recognize differences later when you assist an unhealthy person.

Make sure everyone has the chance to act as the Emergency Responder. Alter circumstances as directed by your instructor.

Secondary Care Skill # 3
Bandaging

Your Goal:

Demonstrate how to bandage a foot, leg, hand or arm using roller bandages and triangular bandages.

Key Points

- Use this skill to determine what first aid may be needed in the event of any injury – especially if Emergency Medical Service is either delayed or unavailable.

- Remember to stop, think, act – assess scene and alert EMS if necessary.

- Use barriers appropriately.

- Perform a patient responsiveness check by giving the responder statement.

- Perform a primary assessment and monitor and treat the patient's *lifeline* if needed.

- Perform an injury assessment.

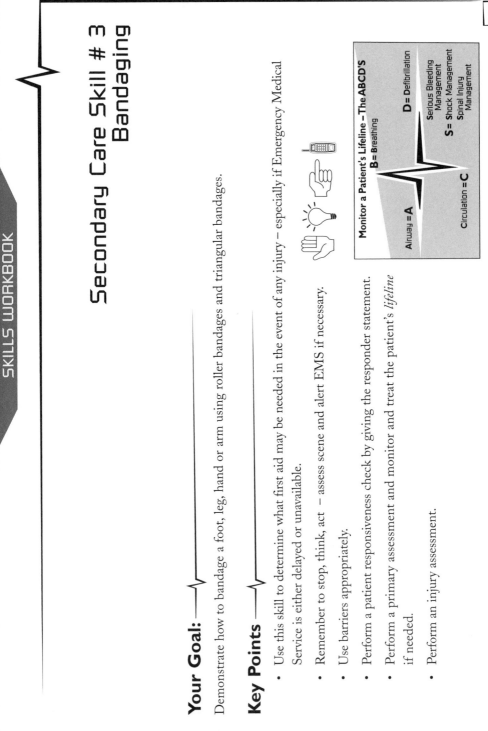

Monitor a Patient's Lifeline – The ABCD'S

B = Breathing

Airway = A

D = Defibrillation

Serious Bleeding Management

S = Shock Management

Spinal Injury Management

Circulation = C

- A first aid kit may include several different types of bandages including triangular bandages, adhesive strips, conforming bandages, gauze rollers (nonelastic cotton) and elastic rollers.

- Choose the best bandage based on the injury or make the best use of whatever is available.

How It's Done

1. Put on gloves.

2. Apply bandage directly over a sterile dressing covering wound.

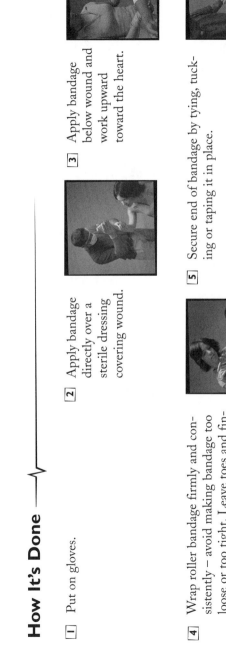

3. Apply bandage below wound and work upward toward the heart.

4. Wrap roller bandage firmly and consistently – avoid making bandage too loose or too tight. Leave toes and fingers exposed to check circulation.

5. Secure end of bandage by tying, tucking or taping it in place.

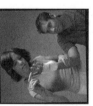

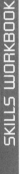

6 When bandaging the foot, secure bandage by wrapping it around the ankle several times then back over injury site on the foot.

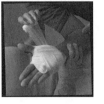

7 When bandaging hand, secure bandage by wrapping it over the thumb and around the wrist.

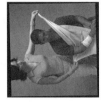

8 If elbow is involved, bandage below and above the joint to stabilize injury site.

9 If the knee is involved, bandage below and above the joint to stabilize the injury.

10 If there is an impaled object, bandage the object in place, do not remove.

Using Triangular Bandages

1 Use triangular bandages to support injuries of the upper arm, ribs or shoulder.

2 Place top of the triangular bandage over the shoulder.

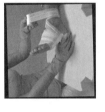

3 Bend arm at the elbow, bring forearm across the chest and over the bandage.

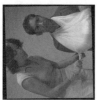

4 Bring lower end of the bandage over the opposite shoulder and tie off at the back of the neck.

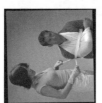

5 Tie off triangular bandage at the patient's elbow, locking the arm in the sling.

6 Support hand, but leave the fingers exposed. Look for color of tissue in fingernails and toenails.

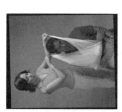

7 When broken ribs are suspected, use a second triangular bandage to hold the arm against the injured side of the chest. Simply tie bandage over the sling and around the chest.

Try It ⚡

In your practice group, practice bandaging a leg or arm using a roller bandage, then use a triangular bandage to make an arm sling. Vary the wound sites – your instructor will direct you. Remember, you only bandage wounds if EMS is either delayed or unavailable.

One person is the guide, reading the steps, one is the patient, while the other is the Emergency Responder. Make sure everyone has the chance to act as the Emergency Responder. Alter circumstances as directed by your instructor.

Secondary Care Skill # 4
Splinting for Dislocations and Fractures

Your Goal

Demonstrate how to apply a splint to a dislocation or fracture.

Key Points

- Use this skill to determine what first aid may be needed in the event of any injury – especially if Emergency Medical Service is either delayed or unavailable.

- Remember to stop, think, then act – assess scene and alert EMS if necessary.

- Use barriers appropriately.

- Perform a patient responsiveness check by giving the responder statement.

- Perform a primary assessment.

- Perform an injury assessment.

Monitor a Patient's Lifeline – The ABCD'S

Airway = **A**

B = Breathing

Circulation = **C**

D = Defibrillation

Serious Bleeding Management

S = Shock Management

Spinal Injury Management

2.68

- Use splinting to protect and immobilize a fractured, dislocated, sprained or strained body part.

- Splints may include a variety of rigid devices including commercial splints or improvised splints (rolled newspapers or magazines, heavy cardboard, padded board, etc.). You may also secure the injured part to an uninjured body part (e.g., injured finger to an uninjured finger; injured arm to the chest, etc.).

- Splint the injury in the position found. Do not try to straighten. Try to minimize movement of the extremity until you complete splinting.

- If available, place splint materials on both sides of the injury site. This prevents rotation of the injured extremity and prevents the bones from touching if two or more bones are involved.

- Splint only if you can do so without causing more discomfort and pain to the patient.

How It's Done

1. Choose a splint long enough to immobilize joints above and below the injury.

2. When using rigid splints, apply ample padding between splint and the injury. Add padding to the natural body hollows as well.

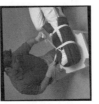

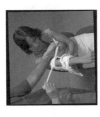

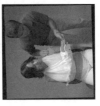

3 Bandage splint in place by using a roller bandage, a triangular bandage, an elastic bandage, adhesive tape or other available materials.

4 Always check circulation before and after splinting. If pulse is absent, loosen the splint until the pulse returns. To do this look for color of tissue in fingernails and toenails.

5 If the fracture is in the upper arm, place arm in sling after splinting.

Try It ⎯⎯ In your practice group, practice splinting a leg or arm. Try a variety of instructor-supplied splinting material. Be resourceful and use possible splinting material found around you.

One person is the guide, reading the steps, one is the patient, while the other is the Emergency Responder. Make sure everyone has the chance to act as the Emergency Responder. Alter circumstances as directed by your instructor.

Three
Emergency Reference

Emergency Reference Table of Contents
Alphabetical Order

EFR Reference

Assembling a First Aid Kit

Build a well-stocked first aid kit using these items:

- Durable noncorrosive case
- *Emergency First Response Participant Manual* – used as reference.
- Emergency phone numbers/coins/phone card – used in an emergency to assist with remembering important contact information
- Gloves – to protect rescuer against bloodborne pathogens
- Ventilation barriers – used to protect rescuer against disease transmission
- Large absorbent dressings; various sizes – used to help stop bleeding
- Sterile gauze pads; various sizes – used to help stop bleeding and dress wounds
- Clinging rolled bandages; various sizes – used to dress wounds
- Adhesive bandages; various sizes – used to dress wounds
- Adhesive tape – used to dress wounds
- Nonadherent, dry pads – used to dress burn wounds
- Triangular bandages – used to immobilize dislocations and fractures
- Sterile cotton – used to dress wounds
- Cotton tipped swabs – used to clean wounds
- Bandage scissors – used to cut bandages and patient apparel

Protect Yourself and Others

Where possible (for maximum protection), when attending to an injured or ill patient:

- Use gloves
- Use ventilation masks or shields
- Use eye or face shields; including eyeglasses or sunglasses, goggles and face masks.
- Always wash your hands or any other area exposed to body fluids with antibacterial soap and water. Scrub vigorously, creating lots of lather. If water is not available, use antibacterial wipes or cleansing liquids.

- Tongue depressors – to check vital signs during illness assessment; could also be used as splinting material for finger dislocations and fractures
- Tweezers – to assist in removing foreign material
- Needle – to assist in removing foreign material
- Safety pins – to attach and secure bandages
- Penlight – for light and to use as an examination tool
- Oral thermometer – to measure temperature as a vital sign
- Squeeze bottle of water – for hydration and patients with heat stroke; burns, eye or wound wash
- Splints – to immobilize dislocations and fractures
- Emergency blanket – for warmth; to cover patients with shock
- Cold packs – for bruises, strains, sprains, eye injuries, stings and dislocations and fractures
- Hot packs – for venomous bites and stings
- Vinegar – to neutralize stinging cells of jellyfish
- Plastic bags – use to dispose of gloves and medical waste; may be used in lieu of actual gloves as a barrier
- Small paper cups – for drinking and to cover eye injuries
- Denatured alcohol – for disinfectant, not to be used on wounds
- Antibacterial soap – to clean wounds
- Antiseptic solution or wipes – for wounds
- Antibiotic ointment – for wounds
- Hydrocortisone ointment – for stings or irritations
- Aspirin and nonaspirin pain relievers – to reduce swelling and patient discomfort
- Antihistamine tablets – for allergic reactions
- Sugar packets, candy or fruit juice – for low blood sugar patients
- Activated charcoal – for poisoning

Primary Care

One Rescuer, Adult CPR

1. **STOP**– Assess and observe scene.

2. **THINK** – Consider your safety and form action plan.

3. **ACT** – Check responsiveness.

4. **ALERT** EMS.

5. Open **AIRWAY** using head tilt-chin lift maneuver (head or neck trauma not suspected) or chin lift maneuver (head or neck trauma suspected).

6. Look, listen and feel for **BREATHING.**

7. No *breathing* – position patient on back and remove obvious obstructions from mouth.

8. Place ventilation barrier over patient's mouth and/or nose.

9. Give two slow and effective rescue **BREATHS.**

10. Check for signs of **CIRCULATION.**

11. No *heartbeat* – locate compression site and position yourself directly over patient.

12. Perform 15 **CHEST COMPRESSIONS** at a rate of 100 compressions per minute. Count One and Two and Three and Four.. etc. up to 15.

13. Administer two rescue breaths. Continue with cycles of 15 compressions and two rescue breaths.

14. After one minute, check for signs of circulation. If still absent, continue CPR.

15. **DEFIBRILLATION** by EMS or Automated External Defibrillator (AED).

16. Manage **Serious** bleeding, **Shock** and **Spinal** injury.

Rescue Breathing – Child (1 – 8 years old)

1. **STOP**– Assess and observe scene.

2. **THINK** – Consider your safety and form action plan.

3. **ACT** – Check responsiveness and send someone to **ALERT** EMS. If you are is alone or the child was rescued from the water, provide immediate rescue breathing and other steps of CPR for one minute before phoning EMS.

4. Open **AIRWAY** using head tilt –chin lift maneuver (head or neck trauma not suspected) or chin lift maneuver (head or neck trauma suspected).

5. Look, listen and feel for **BREATHING**.

6. No *breathing* – position child on back and remove obvious obstructions from mouth.

7. Position ventilation barrier (as appropriate), seal your mouth over child's mouth and pinch nose.

8. Give two slow and effective rescue **BREATHS**.

9. Check for signs of **CIRCULATION**.

10. *Circulation present* – Provide one rescue breath every three seconds (20 per minute.)

11. After one minute, check for signs of breathing and circulation. If breathing is still absent, continue rescue breathing. If circulation is absent, begin CPR.

One Rescuer, Child CPR (1 – 8 years old)

1. After two initial rescue **BREATHS**, check for signs of **CIRCULATION**.

2. *No heartbeat* – locate compression site by following lowest rib upward until you reach the point where ribs meet in the center. Feel for a notch on lower half of sternum and place your middle and index finger on notch. Place the heel of the other hand next to the fingers.

3. Using one arm, perform five **CHEST COMPRESSIONS** at a rate of 100 compressions per minute.

4. Administer one effective rescue breath for every five compressions.

5. After one minute, check for signs of circulation. If still absent, continue CPR.

6. **DEFIBRILLATION** by EMS or Automated External Defibrillator (AED). Remember: Child must be eight years old and weigh more than 25 kilograms/55 pounds to use AED.

Rescue Breathing – Infant (less than 1 year old)

1. **STOP** – Assess and observe scene.

2. **THINK** – Consider your safety and form action plan.

3. **ACT** – Check responsiveness and send someone to **ALERT** EMS. If you are alone or the infant was rescued from the water, provide immediate rescue breathing and other steps of CPR before phoning EMS. Open **AIRWAY** using head tilt–chin lift maneuver (head or neck trauma not suspected) or chin lift maneuver (head or neck trauma suspected).

4. Look, listen and feel for **BREATHING**.

5. *No breathing* – position infant on back and remove obvious obstructions from mouth.

6. Seal your mouth over infant's mouth and nose, if possible. Use ventilation barrier as appropriate.

7. Give two slow, effective and gentle rescue **BREATHS** – puffs of air just enough to make the chest rise.

8. Check for signs of **CIRCULATION**.

9. *Circulation present* – Provide one rescue breath every three seconds (20 per minute).

10. After one minute, check for signs of breathing and circulation. If breathing is still absent, continue rescue breathing.

One Rescuer, Infant CPR (less than 1 year old)

1. After two initial rescue **BREATHS**, check for signs of **CIRCULATION**.

2. *No heartbeat* – locate compression site by drawing an imaginary line from nipple to nipple and placing your index finger on the line in the middle of chest. Place two fingers just below line. Lift the index finger and start compressions with the two fingers on chest.

3. Perform five **CHEST COMPRESSIONS** at a rate of 100 compressions per minute.

4. Administer one effective rescue breath for every five compressions.

5. After one minute, check for signs of circulation. If still absent, continue CPR.

Infant Choking

1. **STOP** – *Is the infant choking?*

2. **THINK** – *Is the airway completely blocked?*

3. **ACT** – Send someone to **ALERT** EMS.

4. Place infant's stomach on your forearm. Support infant's head by placing jaw on your fingers.

5. With infant's head slightly lower than the body, deliver five forceful **BACK BLOWS** between shoulder blades with heel of your hand. If object is not dislodged, support infant's head while keeping spine straight and turn infant over.

6. Locate chest compression site. (Draw a line from nipple to nipple and place your index finger on the line in middle of chest. Place two fingers just below the line. Lift your index finger.)

7. With infant's head lower than body, provide five quick **CHEST COMPRESSIONS**.

8. If object is not dislodged, repeat back blows and chest compressions. Continue until object is dislodged or infant becomes unresponsive.

9. If infant becomes unresponsive, begin CPR. If alone, after one minute, alert EMS, then continue care.

Injury First Aid

Injury Assessment

1. **STOP**– Assess and observe scene.

2. **THINK** – Consider your safety and form action plan.

3. **ACT** – Check responsiveness and **ALERT** EMS.

4. Perform a primary assessment and monitor patient's *lifeline* – **ABCD'S.**

5. Explain what you'll be doing during assessment to the patient.

6. Stabilize patient's head and neck, instructing patient to answer verbally.

7. Begin with head – gently run fingers over forehead, cheeks and chin, feeling for deformities.

8. Check ears and nose for blood or fluid.

9. Place finger in front of patient's eyes and check for smooth tracking. Remind patient to follow finger movement with the eyes and not by turning the head.

10. Check pupils for size, equal to each other and reaction to light.

11. Feel skull and neck for abnormalities.

12. Slide both hands over patient's shoulder blades and gently push against the back with your palms.

13. Move hands outward to the shoulders and gently press inward with your palms.

14. Run two fingers cautiously over the collarbones from shoulders to the center.

15. Stabilize shoulder and gently feel with hands and fingers the upper arm, elbow and wrist. Feel for swelling, hardness, tissue softness, points of tenderness or deformities. Ask the patient to wiggle fingers and squeeze your hand. Repeat on the other arm.

16. Place your hands, palms in, on each side of patient's ribcage and gently push inward.

17. Reach around and feel along spinal column from each side without moving patient.

18. Gently push on patient's abdomen – right and left side, above and below navel.

19. Move hands over patient's hip bones, palms in, and gently push inward.

20. Feel the patient's upper leg, knee, lower leg and ankle with hands and fingers. Feel for swelling, hardness, tissue softness, points of tenderness or deformities. Ask the patient to wiggle toes and press the sole of the foot against your hand. Repeat on the other leg.

21. Note areas of pain or abnormality to report to EMS personnel.

22. Continue to monitor patient's *lifeline.*

23. Avoid giving injured patient anything to eat or drink as the patient may need surgery.

Dislocations and Fractures

Out-of-socket joints, cracked, broken, separated and shattered bones

Important Information

- *Dislocations occur when a great deal of pressure is placed on a joint. The patient's joint appears deformed and the injury is very painful.*

- *Suspect a fracture if, after a fall or blow a limb appears to be in an unnatural position, is unusable, swells or bruises rapidly or is extremely painful at a specific point.*

- *Only splint an injury if EMS care or transport to a medical facility is delayed and if you can do so without causing more discomfort and pain to patient.*

- *All dislocations and fractures need professional medical attention.*

Patient Care

1. **STOP**– Assess and observe scene.

2. **THINK** – Consider your safety and form action plan.

3. **ACT** – Check responsiveness and **ALERT** EMS, as appropriate.

4. For patient involved in a major fall, collision or blow, conduct injury assessment to determine extent of all injuries besides obvious dislocation or fracture.

5. If EMS is delayed or unavailable prepare patient for transport. Choose a splint that is long enough to immobilize the bones above and below the unstable joint.

6. Splint injury in position found. Do not try to straighten. Minimize movement while splinting.

7. Bandage splint in place by using a triangle bandage or other available materials.

8. Fractured fingers and toes may be taped to adjacent fingers or toes for support.

9. Check circulation before and after splinting. Loosen splint if it interferes with circulation.

10. For closed fractures or dislocation, apply cold compress to area during transport to reduce swelling.

Minor Cuts, Scrapes and Bruises

Non life threatening wounds – lacerations, scratches, abrasions, gashes, punctures and bumps.

Important Information

- *Deep cuts or punctures need to be treated by a medical professional.*

- *Patients with wounds that do not stop bleeding with direct pressure or pressure points need immediate EMS care.*

Patient Care – Cuts and Scrapes

1. Wear gloves and other barriers to protect yourself and patient from disease transmission.
2. If necessary, control bleeding with direct pressure.
3. Thoroughly wash wound with water to remove all dirt and particles.
4. Cover wound with a nonadhesive dressing and bandage securely.
5. Check wound daily for signs of infection – redness, tenderness or presence of pus (yellowish or greenish fluid at wound site).

Patient Care – Bruises

1. Apply cold compress to injured area as soon as possible.
2. Elevate affected area above the heart, if possible.

Dental Injury

Fractured jaw, loose tooth, broken tooth, dislodged tooth, bitten lip or tongue.

Important Information

- *Treat dental injuries resulting from trauma to the head, neck, face or mouth as medical emergencies. Follow primary and secondary care procedures.*
- *Send patient to a dentist for treatment when dental injuries are due to wear and tear, or minor mishaps. Provide secondary care.*

Patient Care – Dislodged Tooth

1. Wear gloves to protect yourself and patient from disease transmission.

2. Locate dislodged tooth. Do not touch the root.

3. Hold tooth by crown and rinse gently with saline solution, milk or water.

4. Keep tooth moist in saline solution, milk or water while transporting to dentist.

5. If unable to get to dentist within 60 minutes, reimplant tooth into socket as soon as possible. Teeth reimplanted within 30 to 60 minutes have a good chance of reattaching to socket.

6. Encourage patient to follow up with continued dental care.

Strains and Sprains

— Injured, stretched or torn muscles, tendons and ligaments

Important Information

- *General treatment involves RICE – Rest, Ice, Compression and Elevation for the first 72 hours after injury.*

- *Patients should consult a medical professional to determine the extent of the injury and to ensure no bones are broken.*

Patient Care

1. REST – take stress off injured area and avoid use as much as possible.

2. ICE – apply cold compress to injured area for up to 20 minutes. Repeat icing at least four times a day.

3. **COMPRESSION** – wrap area with elastic bandage.

4. **ELEVATE** – raise injured area above the heart as much as possible.

5. If patient must use injured area, tape or splint to provide stability and prevent further injury.

6. Anti-inflammatory tablets or pain relievers may reduce pain and inflammation.

7. Encourage patient to follow up with a doctor.

Eye Injuries

Cuts, penetrations, blows, chemical splashes and irritants

Important Information

- *Treat eye injuries that result from trauma to the head or face as medical emergencies. Follow primary and secondary care procedures.*

- *Never apply pressure to the eye and be careful not to rub it.*

- *If patient wears contact lenses, remove them only if it will not cause further damage to the eye.*

- *Encourage patients with any eye soreness or irritation to see an eye specialist for treatment as soon as possible. Provide secondary care.*

- *Encourage patient to keep calm. Increased activity and blood pressure can cause important eye fluids to leak causing further harm to the eye.*

Patient Care – Cuts and Penetrations to Eye

1. STOP– Assess and observe scene.
2. THINK – Consider your safety and form action plan.
3. ACT – Check responsiveness and **ALERT** EMS.
4. Perform a primary assessment and monitor patient's *lifeline* – **ABCD'S.**
5. Apply a sterile dressing and lightly bandage the eye.
6. If penetrating object protrudes from eye, place a small paper cup over eye and bandage in place. Do NOT remove object.
7. Consider covering both eyes to deter patient from moving injured eye.
8. Continue to monitor patient's *lifeline* until EMS arrives.

Patient Care – Blow to Eye

1. STOP– Assess and observe scene.
2. THINK – Consider your safety and form action plan.
3. ACT – Check responsiveness and **ALERT** EMS, as appropriate.
4. Perform a primary assessment and monitor patient's *lifeline* – **ABCD'S.**
5. Apply cold compresses for 15 minutes.
6. If EMS is not called, encourage patient to see eye specialist as soon as possible.

Patient Care – Chemical Splashes in the Eye

1. STOP– Assess and observe scene.
2. THINK – Consider your safety and form action plan.
3. ACT – Check responsiveness and **ALERT** EMS, as appropriate.

[4] Perform a primary assessment and monitor patient's *lifeline* – ABCD'S.

[5] Immediately flush eye with water until EMS arrives or for a minimum of 15 minutes.

[6] Open eye as wide as possible and ask patient to roll eye to aid flushing.

[7] If EMS is delayed, continue flushing, Do not bandage eye.

Patient Care — Irritants in the Eye

[1] Wear gloves to protect yourself and patient from disease transmission.

[2] Inspect eye and attempt to locate irritant.

[3] Either you or the patient should lift the upper lid and gently pull it down over lower eye lashes.

[4] Encourage patient to blink and let tears wash irritant away.

[5] If irritant remains, flush the eye with a gentle stream of water.

[6] If irritant remains, carefully attempt to dislodge it with a sterile moistened cloth.

[7] If irritant remains, have patient seek treatment from an eye specialist.

Electrical Injury

Electric shock, electrocution and electrical burns

Important Information

- *Any contact with electricity can cause life threatening injuries such as cardiopulmonary arrest, deep burns and internal tissue damage.*

- *Treat electrical shock that alters the patient's consciousness, results in burns or is associated with collisions or falls as medical emergencies. Follow primary and secondary care procedures.*

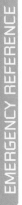

- *Any injury caused by electric shock should be examined by a medical professional.*

Patient Care

1 **STOP**– Assess and observe scene – *Is patient still in contact with electricity?*

2 **THINK** – Consider your safety and form action plan – *Make sure electricity is off.*

3 **ACT** – Check responsiveness and **ALERT** EMS, as appropriate.

4 Perform a primary assessment

5 Monitor patient's *lifeline* and attend to **ABCD'S**

6 If patient is responsive, perform a secondary assessment – look for burns.

7 Treat burns by flushing with cool water until EMS arrives. (See *Burns* for more information)

8 If EMS is not called, encourage patient to see a doctor.

Temperature-Related Injuries

Burns

Thermal, chemical and electrical burns.

Important Information

- *First-degree burns affect only the outer skin layer. The skin is red, slightly swollen and painful to touch. Sunburn usually falls into this category.*

- *Second-degree burns go into the second skin layer and appear as blisters on red, splotchy skin.*

- *Third-degree burns involve all layers of the skin – even underlying tissue. These serious burns are often painless due to nerve destruction. They appear as charred black or dry and white areas.*

- *Treat any large burn on the face, hands, feet, groin, buttocks or a major joint as a medical emergency. Follow primary and secondary care procedures.*

- *Never put ice, butter, grease, ointments, creams or oils on a burn.*

Patient Care – Major Burns
(third-degree or second-degree larger than 5-7.5 centimetres/2-3 inches)

1. **STOP** – Assess and observe scene – *Where is the heat source?*

2. **THINK** – Consider your safety and form action plan – *Is patient's clothing or surroundings still on fire or hot?*

3. **ACT** – Check responsiveness and **ALERT EMS**.

4. Perform a primary assessment and monitor the patient's *lifeline* – ABCD'S.

5. If patient is responsive, perform secondary assessment to determine extent of burns.

6. Cover burns with cool, moist sterile bandage or clean cloth.

7. For finger or toe burns, remove jewelry and separate with dry, sterile, nonadhesive dressings.

8. Continue to monitor patient's *lifeline* until EMS arrives – manage shock.

Patient Care – Minor Burns (first degree and small second-degree)

1. Wear gloves to protect yourself and patient from disease transmission.

2. Flush or soak burn in cool water for at least five minutes.

3. Cover area with a sterile bandage.

4 Skin lotions may help prevent drying and provide comfort.

5 Pain relievers may reduce pain and inflammation.

6 Check burn daily for signs of infection – redness, tenderness or presence of pus (yellowish or greenish fluid at wound site).

Patient Care – Chemical Burn

1 **STOP**– Assess and observe scene – *What and where are chemicals?*

2 **THINK** – Consider your safety and form action plan – *How can you avoid chemical contact?*

3 **ACT** – Check responsiveness and **ALERT** EMS, as appropriate.

4 Perform a primary assessment and monitor the patient's *lifeline* – **ABCD'S**.

5 For liquid chemicals, flush skin surface with cool, running water for at least 20 minutes.

6 For powder chemicals, brush off skin before flushing with water.

7 Cover burn with a dry, sterile dressing or a clean cloth.

8 If EMS is not called, encourage patient to see a doctor.

Hypothermia

Severe hypothermia – body temperature below 32°Celsius (C)/90°Fahrenheit (F)
Mild hypothermia – body temperature lowered to 34°Celsius (C)/93°Fahrenheit (F)

Important Information

- *A patient suffering from severe hypothermia may be disoriented, confused, uncoordinated or completely unresponsive.*

- *A patient suffering from mild hypothermia may be conscious and alert, yet shivering and displaying slightly impaired coordination.*

- *Treat hypothermia that alters the patient's consciousness or impairs coordination as a medical emergency. Follow primary care procedures.*
- *A severely hypothermic patient may be breathing or have a pulse at such a low rate and intensity that it is difficult to detect. Therefore, resuscitation attempts should never be abandoned until the patient has been rewarmed.*

Patient Care – Severe Hypothermia

1. **STOP**– Assess and observe scene – *Has patient been exposed to a cold environment?*
2. **THINK** – Consider your safety and form action plan – *Is a warm, dry area nearby?*
3. **ACT** – Check responsiveness and **ALERT** EMS.
4. Perform a primary assessment and monitor the patient's *lifeline* – **ABCD'S.**
5. Do not move patient unless necessary to prevent further heat loss. Handling may cause irregular heartbeat.
6. Remove wet clothing without jostling patient. Cover patient with warm blankets or thick clothing.
7. Continue to monitor patient's *lifeline* until EMS arrives.

Patient Care – Mild Hypothermia

1. Move patient to a warm and dry sheltered area and wrap in warm blankets or clothes.
2. If patient is wet, provide with dry clothing.
3. Give warm, nonalcoholic, noncaffeinated drinks.
4. Continue to support patient until completely rewarmed.

Frostbite

Frostnip, superficial and deep frostbite

Important Information

- *Frostbite occurs when an area of the body freezes and ice crystals form within cells.*

- *Frostnip is the first stage that affects the surface skin. The skin becomes red, painful and may itch.*

- *Superficial frostbite affects skin layers, but not the soft tissue below. The skin becomes hard and white.*

- *Deep frostbite affects entire tissue layers including muscles, tendons, blood vessels, and nerves. The area may be white, deep purple or red with blisters, and feel hard and woody.*

- *Treat frostbite as a medical emergency. Follow primary and secondary care procedures.*

Patient Care

1. **STOP**– Assess and observe scene – *Has patient been exposed to a cold environment?*

2. **THINK** – Consider your safety and form action plan – *Is a warm, dry area nearby?*

3. **ACT** – Check responsiveness and **ALERT** EMS.

4. Perform a primary and secondary assessment. Monitor the patient's *lifeline* – **ABCD'S.**

5. Move patient to a warm and dry sheltered area.

6. Begin to warm affected areas with your body heat or by immersing in warm (not hot) water. Rescuer should check the water to make sure it is only warm. Warm slowly.

7. Do not rub or massage frostbitten areas. Note that rewarming may be very painful.

8. Continue to monitor patient's *lifeline* until EMS arrives.

Heat Stroke and Exhaustion

Heat stroke – body temperature higher than 40°C/104°F
Heat exhaustion – fluid loss and body temperature up to 40°C/104°F

Important Information

- *Heat stroke occurs when the body's temperature control system fails and body temperature rises dangerously high. It is a life threatening condition.*

- *Patients with heat stroke may have hot, dry, flushed skin, rapid pulse and be disoriented, confused or unconscious.*

- *Treat heat stroke as a medical emergency. Follow primary care procedures.*

- *Heat exhaustion occurs when fluid intake does not compensate for perspiration loss.*

- *Patients with heat exhaustion may have cool and clammy skin, weak pulse and complain of nausea, dizziness, weakness and anxiety.*

Patient Care – Heat Stroke

1. **STOP** – Assess and observe scene – *Has patient been exposed to a hot environment?*
2. **THINK** – Consider your safety and form action plan – *Is a cool, shady area nearby?*
3. **ACT** – Check responsiveness and **ALERT EMS.**
4. Perform a primary assessment. Monitor the patient's *lifeline* – **ABCD'S.**
5. Move patient to a cool, shady area.
6. Immediately cool patient by spraying or sponging with cool water.
7. Cover patient with wet cloth and continue to monitor patient's *lifeline* until EMS arrives.

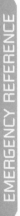

Patient Care – Heat Exhaustion

1 Move patient to cool location.

2 Urge patient to lie down and elevate legs.

3 Provide patient with cool water or an electrolyte-containing beverage to drink every few minutes.

4 Cool patient by misting with water and fanning.

5 Continue to support patient until completely cooled.

6 If EMS is not called, encourage patient to see a doctor.

Illness First Aid

Illness Assessment

Illness Assessment – An illness is an *unhealthy condition of the body*. An illness assessment helps you identify and report medical problems that affect a patient's health and may aid in the patient's treatment.

Important Information

- *Use this skill to determine what first aid may be needed in the event that Emergency Medical Service is either delayed or unavailable.*

- *Only perform illness assessments on conscious, responsive patients.*

- *When giving information to EMS personnel, avoid using the word normal. Provide measured rates per minute and descriptive terminology.*

Patient Care

1. **STOP** – Assess and observe scene.
2. **THINK** – Consider your safety and form action plan.
3. **ACT** – Check responsiveness.
4. **ALERT** EMS.

- Find a paper and a pen/pencil to record illness assessment information. Use Illness Assessment Record Sheet at the end of this section.
- If possible, have someone else record information.
- Put on gloves.

SAMPLE – Signs and Symptoms

5. Ask how patient is feeling and what occurred immediately before the onset of illness. Questions may include:

   ❯ How do you feel now?
   ❯ What were you doing when you began to feel ill?
   ❯ When did the first symptoms occur?
   ❯ Where were you when the first symptoms occurred?

Finding Pulse Rate

6. To find pulse rate using the carotid artery:

   ❯ Locate the patient's adam's apple with the index and middle fingers of one hand.
   ❯ Slide the fingers down into the groove of the neck on the side closest to you.

✓ If you can't find the pulse on the side closest to you, move to the opposite side.

✓ Never try to feel the carotid pulse on both sides at the same time.

✓ Count the number of beats in 30 seconds and multiply by two to determine the heartbeats per minute.

7 To find pulse rate using the radial artery:

✓ Locate artery on patient's wrist, thumb side of hand.

✓ Slide two or three fingers into the groove of the wrist immediately below hand on the thumb side.

Do not use your thumb when taking a radial pulse.

✓ Count the number of beats in 30 seconds and multiply by two to determine the heartbeats per minute.

✓ Determine whether the pulse may be described as rapid, strong or weak.

Checking Respiration

8 Look for signs and symptoms of respiratory distress, including:

✓ Wheezing, gurgling or high-pitched noises when the patient breathes.

✓ Patient complains of shortness of breath or feeling dizzy or lightheaded.

✓ Patient complains of pain in the chest and numbness or tingling in arms or legs.

9 Evaluate breathing by either:

✓ Placing a hand on patient's abdomen or watch chest rise and fall.

✓ Counting patient's respiration for 30 seconds and multiplying by two to determine respiratory rate.

10 Determine whether respiration may be described as fast, slow, labored, wheezing or gasping.

Checking temperature and moisture

11 Feel patient's forehead or cheek with the back of your hand. Compare with your own temperature using your other hand on your forehead. Verify if the patient has perhaps been doing physical exercise.

12 Determine whether the skin is warm, hot, cool, moist, clammy, etc.

Determining Color

13 Look for apparent skin color changes that may be described as extremely pale, ashen (grey), red, blue, yellowish or black-and-blue blotches.

14 If the patient has dark skin, check for color changes on the nailbeds, lips, gums, tongue, palms, whites of the eyes, and ear lobes.

sAMPLE – Allergies

15 Ask if patient is allergic to anything – food, drugs, airborne matter, etc.

16 Ask if the patient has ingested or taken anything the patient may be allergic to.

saMPLE – Medications

17 Ask if patient takes medication for a medical condition. Questions may include:

> Do you take medication?
> If yes, what type of medication do you take?
> Did you take medication today?
> How much medication did you take and when?

18 If possible, collect all medication to give to EMS personnel and/or get name of the doctor who prescribed the medication.

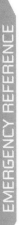

SAMPLE – PreExisting Medical Conditions

19 Ask if patient has a preexisting medical condition (e.g., heart condition, diabetes, asthma, epilepsy, etc.)

SAMPLE – Last Meal

20 Ask when patient last had a meal and what patient ate.

SAMPLE – Events

21 Ask patient about or note events leading up to illness.

22 Provide EMS personnel with information and measured breathing and pulse rates.

Heart Attack
Important Information

- *The most common heart attack symptom is chest pain (angina) accompanied by pressure or squeezing in the center of the chest that lasts for several minutes, or is intermittent and reoccurring.*

- *Heart attack pain may spread to the shoulders, neck or arms. The patient may sweat or faint or complain of nausea, shortness of breath and dizziness.*

- *Patient may deny that chest discomfort is serious enough for emergency medical care. Use your judgment and don't delay alerting EMS if you suspect a heart attack.*

Patient Care

1. **STOP** – Assess and observe scene.

2. **THINK** – Consider your safety and form action plan.

3. **ACT** – Check responsiveness, look for medical alert tag and **ALERT** EMS.

4. Perform a primary assessment and monitor patient's *lifeline* – **ABCD'S.**

5. For an unresponsive patient, perform CPR as necessary.

6. For a responsive patient, conduct an illness assessment. If the patient has angina (chest pains) and nitroglycerin is available, assist patient in taking his medication as prescribed. If so directed by Emergency Medical Services personnel, you may administer aspirin to the patient.

7. Help patient into a comfortable position and loosen tight fitting clothes, collars, etc.

8. Continue to monitor patient's *lifeline* until EMS arrives. Consider administering oxygen if available.

Stroke
Important Information

- *Strokes occur when a blood vessel in the brain is blocked or ruptures depriving brain tissue of oxygen. Think of a stroke as a brain attack (versus a heart attack). Stroke is a clog in the brain as opposed to a clog in the heart. There are methods for unclogging strokes in a hospital's emergency room. Remember to alert EMS immediately for a suspected stroke patient.*

- *Patients having a stroke may complain or have signs of numbness, paralysis or weakness of the face, arm or leg, often just one side, and may have trouble speaking. They may complain of a severe, unexplained headache or decreased vision in one or both eyes.*

- *Treat a stroke as a medical emergency. Follow primary care procedures.*

Patient Care

1. **STOP**– Assess and observe scene.
2. **THINK** – Consider your safety and form action plan.
3. **ACT** – Check responsiveness, look for medical alert tag and **ALERT** EMS.
4. Perform a primary assessment and monitor patient's *lifeline* – **ABCD'S**.
5. For a responsive patient, conduct an illness assessment. If the patient has difficulty speaking, reassure the patient and ask yes or no questions.
6. Help patient into a comfortable position.
7. Continue to monitor patient's *lifeline* until EMS arrives.

Diabetic Problems

Low blood sugar – insulin shock, insulin reaction or hypoglycemia
High blood sugar – diabetic coma, diabetic ketoacidosis or hyperglycemia

Important Information

* *An insulin reaction occurs when a person with diabetes receives too much insulin, does not get enough sugar from food or engages in strenuous exercise that quickly decreases blood sugar levels.*

* *Patients suffering from low blood sugar may appear pale, have moist skin and sweat excessively. Patients may complain of a headache and dizziness, and be irritable and confused.*

* *Diabetic ketoacidosis occurs when a person with diabetes does not have enough insulin to control rising blood sugar levels.*

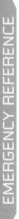

3.28

- Early symptoms of high blood sugar include thirst and frequent urination. Advanced signs and symptoms include drowsiness and confusion, rapid, weak pulse and rapid breathing with a fruity odor on breath. The patient may also have nausea, vomiting, and abdominal pain. Treat advanced cases as a medical emergency.

- Never give a patient insulin or medication – even if the patient asks. When in doubt, always provide the patient with a small snack, meal, sugar, fruit juice, soda or candy. Sugar is crucial for low blood sugar, and won't cause significant harm to a patient with high blood sugar.

Patient Care – Low Blood Sugar

1 **STOP**– Assess and observe scene.

2 **THINK** – Consider your safety and form action plan.

3 **ACT** – Check responsiveness, look for medical alert tag and **ALERT** EMS, as appropriate.

4 Perform a primary assessment. Monitor the patient's *lifeline* – **ABCD'S**.

5 For an unresponsive patient, manage shock until EMS arrives.

6 For a responsive patient, conduct an illness assessment.

7 Quickly provide the patient with a small snack or meal for sustained relief. If sugar, fruit juice, soda or candy are available they can help when nothing else is available.

8 Continue to support patient until signs and symptoms subside – approximately 15 minutes. If patient does not improve, transport to nearest medical facility.

Patient Care – High Blood Sugar

1 **STOP**– Assess and observe scene.

2 **THINK** – Consider your safety and form action plan.

3 ACT – Check responsiveness, look for medical alert tag and **ALERT** EMS.

4 Perform a primary assessment and monitor the patient's *lifeline* – **ABCD'S.**

5 For an unresponsive patient, manage shock until EMS arrives. If in doubt as to whether the patient has high blood sugar or low blood sugar, always provide the patient with a small snack or meal.

6 For a responsive patient, conduct an illness assessment and monitor the patient's *lifeline* until EMS arrives.

Seizures

Important Information

- *Seizures or convulsions may result from epilepsy, heat stroke, poisoning, hypoglycemia, high fever in children, brain injury, stroke or electric shock.*

- *Treat a seizure as a medical emergency when the patient does not have epilepsy or a seizure disorder; if the seizure lasts for more than five minutes, has a series of seizures or there are associated injuries and illnesses that require care. Follow primary care procedures.*

Patient Care

1 STOP– Assess and observe scene – *Does the patient have a seizure disorder?*

2 THINK – Consider safety and form action plan – *Are there harmful objects near the patient?*

3 ACT – Check responsiveness, look for medical alert tag and **ALERT** EMS, as appropriate.

4 During seizure, attempt to cushion patient's head and move objects out of the way, but do not restrain patient. Protect the patient.

5 After seizure, conduct primary assessment. Place breathing patient in recovery position.

6 For patient with a seizure disorder, support and reassure patient until recovered.

7 For patient with no history of seizures or if patient is injured during seizure, continue to monitor the patient's *lifeline* until EMS arrives.

Allergic Reactions

— Severe reaction – anaphylaxis or anaphylactic shock

Important Information

- *Severe reactions occur rapidly – usually immediately after the patient eats, is bitten by an insect or takes medication.*

- *Patients having severe allergic reactions may have hives, wheezing, chest tightness, stomach pain and complain of nausea, difficulty breathing and swallowing due to swollen throat tissue. Their blood pressure may drop, leading to dizziness and fainting.*

- *Treat a severe allergic reaction as a medical emergency and follow primary care procedures.*

- *Mild allergic reactions include sneezing, itchy eyes, runny nose and skin rashes. Mild allergies are not life threatening and are usually controlled by antihistamines.*

Patient Care – Allergic Reaction; Anaphylaxis

1 **STOP** – Assess and observe scene – *Was patient stung? Eating?*

2 **THINK** – Consider your safety and form action plan – *Is epinephrine available?*

3 **ACT** – Check responsiveness, look for medical alert tag and **ALERT** EMS.

4 Perform a primary assessment and monitor patient's *lifeline* – **ABCD'S.**

5 If patient carries an epinephrine kit, help patient use it following included directions. Continue to support patient until EMS arrives.

6 If epinephrine is not available, continue to monitor patient's *lifeline* until EMS arrives. Responsive patients may prefer to sit up for easier breathing.

Poisoning

Ingested Poisons – medications, chemicals, cleaners, solvents, pesticides and plant material
Inhaled Poisons – Carbon monoxide, gases and toxic fumes
Absorbed Poisons – poison ivy, oak or sumac and chemical sprays
Food Poisoning – Ingested poisoning by foods

Important Information

* *Suspect poisoning when a source is nearby or patients state that they've come in contact with toxic substances.*

* *Different chemicals cause different reactions within the body. In general, patients who have ingested poison may have burns or stains around the mouth, excessive salivation, sweating, nausea and tear formation. Their breath may smell like chemicals and they may have difficulty breathing. Vomiting, diarrhea, convulsions, drowsiness and unconsciousness may occur.*

* *Patients who inhale carbon monoxide or other harmful substances may experience headache, dizziness, nausea and chest tightness. They may cough, wheeze and have difficulty breathing. Their skin may become pale, then bluish and nailbeds and lips may appear cherry–red.*

* *In mild cases, patients who absorb poison through their skin may have swelling skin, rash, itching, burning and blisters. Symptoms may be delayed. In more serious cases, patients may also complain of difficulty breathing, fever, headache and weakness.*

- Food poisoning occurs when people eat foods contaminated by bacteria or eat food that is toxic, such as certain mushrooms, fish or shellfish. Symptoms may be delayed and include severe stomach cramps, nausea, vomiting, diarrhea, weakness and general discomfort.

- Treat any suspected ingested or inhaled poisoning, or any poisoning that alters the patient's breathing or consciousness level, as a medical emergency. Follow primary care procedures.

- If possible, contact your local Poison Control Center for directions while waiting for EMS to arrive.

Patient Care – Ingested Poison

1. **STOP**– Assess and observe scene – *Is there a poisonous substance nearby?*

2. **THINK** – Consider your safety and form action plan – *Can the substance harm me?*

3. **ACT** – Check responsiveness and **ALERT** EMS.

4. Perform a primary assessment and monitor patient's *lifeline* – **ABCD'S.**

5. For a responsive patient, conduct an illness assessment –

Keep It Safe – Dos and Don'ts

To avoid accidental poisoning:

DO follow directions and caution labels on chemical products.

DO use safety locks on cabinets and keep harmful substances out of small children's reach.

DO store chemicals, cleaners and medicines in original containers, clearly marked and separated from nonpoisonous items.

DO return chemical products to safe storage after use.

DO know what kind of plants you have in and around the home.

DO wear protective clothing and shields when spraying or handling toxic substances.

DO teach children about poisonous substances.

DO keep your local Poison Control Center number near the phone.

DO keep activated charcoal handy and use it only when instructed by EMS, your doctor or Poison Control Center.

DO NOT mix household cleaning products or other chemicals together.

DO NOT use food containers to store chemical products.

DO NOT call medicine candy.

DO NOT take medications in the dark.

DO NOT eat wild mushrooms or plant leaves, stems, roots or berries unless you are absolutely positive they are nontoxic.

DO NOT eat foods that may be spoiled or prepared in unclean conditions.

gather information about what, when and how much poison was ingested while waiting for EMS to arrive.

6 If available, read label on substance for poisoning instructions and call Poison Control Center for direction.

7 If instructed to induce vomiting, use substance recommended by local Poison Control Center. Save vomitus and gather poison container for EMS personnel.

8 Continue to follow Poison Control Center directions and support patient until EMS arrives.

Patient Care – Inhaled Poison

1 **STOP**– Assess and observe scene – *Is there a poisonous substance or fumes nearby?* Be very cautious of entering enclosed spaces.

2 Remember, some poisonous gases are both odorless and colorless. Emergency Responder safety must be considered at all times. You may have to wait for EMS to arrive with independent breathing equipment to actually assist the patient.

3 **THINK** – Consider your safety and form action plan – *Can the substance harm me?*

4 **ACT** – Check responsiveness and **ALERT** EMS.

5 If necessary, move patient to area with fresh air.

6 Perform a primary assessment and monitor patient's *lifeline* – **ABCD'S**.

7 For a responsive patient, help loosen clothing around the neck and chest for easier breathing. Conduct an illness assessment – gather information about what, when and how much poison was inhaled while waiting for EMS to arrive.

8 Contact local Poison Control Center for direction. If available and permitted, administer emergency oxygen.

9 Continue to support patient until EMS arrives.

Patient Care – Absorbed Poison

1. **STOP**– Assess and observe scene – *Has patient come in contact with a poisonous substance?*
2. **THINK** – Consider your safety and form action plan – *Can the substance harm me?*
3. **ACT** – Check responsiveness and **ALERT** EMS, as appropriate.
4. Conduct an illness assessment – gather information about what, when and how much contact the patient had with poison.
5. Carefully remove contaminated clothing and brush off any poison remaining on skin.
6. Flush area with fresh water and wash skin with soap.
7. For caustic chemical substances or if patient experiences severe symptoms, contact local Poison Control Center for direction.
8. If EMS is not called, encourage patient to see a doctor. Cold compresses may relieve itching.

Patient Care – Food Poisoning

1. **STOP**– Assess and observe scene – *Could the patient have eaten something spoiled, contaminated or harmful?*
2. **THINK** – Consider your safety and form action plan.
3. **ACT** – Check responsiveness and **ALERT** EMS, as appropriate.
4. Conduct an illness assessment – ask what the patient ate.
5. If patient shows signs of a severe allergic reaction, treat appropriately. (See *Allergic Reactions* for more information.) Monitor the patient's *lifeline* until EMS arrives.
6. If patient vomits and has diarrhea, offer fluids to prevent dehydration. Continue to support patient until recovered. Consider saving a sample of expelled body fluids for examination by medical professionals to determine the type of poison.
7. If symptoms are severe, prolonged or get worse, transport patient to a medical facility.

Venomous Bites and Stings

Snake and reptile bites, spider bites, scorpion, bee and ant stings, aquatic life injuries

Important Information

- Suspect a venomous bite or sting when a venomous creature is nearby or patients state that they've been bitten or stung. If possible and safe, get a good look at the creature or capture it for positive identification, however do not take time away from patient care or put yourself at risk.

- Reaction to venom may depend on the patient's size, current health, previous exposure, body chemistry, location of bite or sting and how much venom was injected. Some patients have severe allergic reactions to even minor bites or stings – particularly bee stings. See Allergic Reactions for treatment of anaphylaxis.

- Patients bitten by a venomous snake or reptile may have fang marks along with pain, swelling and skin discoloration at bite site. They may complain of weakness, nausea, difficulty breathing, speaking or swallowing, headache, blurred vision and tingling or numbness around the face or mouth. They may have a rapid pulse, fever, chills and may vomit.

- Patients bitten by a venomous spider may have pain, redness and/or heat at the bite site along with abdominal pain and muscle cramps or twitching, confusion, coma and copious secretion of saliva. The patient may also complain of headaches, nausea, difficulty breathing and dizziness. Profuse sweating and extremity numbness may occur along with tingling around the mouth. Often, symptoms do not occur for more than an hour after a bite.

- Insect bites and stings usually result in pain, redness, itching, and swelling at bite site. Some patients may experience delayed reactions such as fever, painful joints, hives and swollen glands.

- Many aquatic life stings result in burning or sharp pain at the sting site along with swelling and/or red rash and welts. Some patients may experience shock, unconsciousness, respiratory difficulty or arrest, weakness, nausea and vomiting.

- Some bites or stings by venomous creatures result in no venom being injected into the patient and cause only minor irritation. However, because symptoms may be delayed, encourage the patient to seek professional medical followup to prevent future disability.

- Treat any bite or sting by a highly venomous creature as a medical emergency. Follow primary care procedures.

- Treat any bite or sting that produces a deep wound, or alters the patient's breathing or consciousness level, as a medical emergency. Follow primary care procedures.

- If possible, contact your local Poison Control Center for directions while waiting for EMS to arrive.

- For many venomous bites and stings, use pressure immobilization to slow the spread of venom. Technique is pictured below.

Apply a broad, firm bandage over the bite as soon as possible. Keep the bitten area still.

The bandage should be as tight as you would apply to a sprained ankle.

Extend the bandages as high as possible.

Apply a splint to the limb.

Bind it firmly to as much of the limb as possible.

Patient Care – Snake Bites

1. **STOP**– Assess and observe scene – *Is there a venomous snake nearby?* Remember, some snakes may bite more than once. Protect yourself. Treat all snake bites as potentially lethal and manage as listed below.

2. **THINK** – Consider your safety and form action plan – *Can it reach me or the patient?*

3. **ACT** – Check responsiveness and **ALERT** EMS.

4. Perform a primary assessment and monitor patient's *lifeline* – **ABCD'S**.

5. Once EMS is contacted, obtain and follow local medical control directions for field treatment prior to their arrival.

6. In general, keep the patient quiet by having the patient lie down and try to relax.

7. Unless directed by EMS to do otherwise, avoid cleaning the wound as saliva from the snake may assist EMS in identifying the snake.

8. If EMS is delayed or unavailable you must transport patient. Administration of antiveninom is the only effective treatment for poisonous snakebites. Therefore, prompt transport to a medical facility is important. Carry the patient if possible or have the patient walk slowly.

9. Place direct pressure on the wound with a sterile dressing, pad or gloved hand.

10. Next, apply pressure immobilization.

11. Continue to monitor patient's *lifeline* until EMS arrives or during transport.

Patient Care – Spider Bites

1. **STOP**– Assess and observe scene – *Is there a venomous insect nearby?*

2. **THINK** – Consider your safety and form action plan – *Can it reach me or the patient?*

3. **ACT** – Check responsiveness and **ALERT** EMS, as appropriate.

4. Perform a primary assessment and monitor patient's *lifeline* – **ABCD'S**.

5 Once EMS is contacted, obtain and follow local medical control directions for field treatment prior to their arrival.

6 If patient shows signs of a severe allergic reaction, treat appropriately. (See *Allergic Reactions* for more information.) Monitor the patient's *lifeline* until EMS arrives.

7 Reassure and keep patient still and at rest.

8 Depending on the directions from EMS: a) clean the bite area with soap and water or rubbing alcohol, b) apply cold compress to area and elevate or c) apply pressure immobilization.

9 Transport to medical facility as antivenin exists for some spiders.

Patient Care – Insect Stings (scorpion, bee, wasp and ant)

1 **STOP**– Assess and observe scene – *Is there a venomous insect nearby?*

2 **THINK** – Consider your safety and form action plan – *Can it reach me or the patient?*

3 **ACT** – Check responsiveness and **ALERT EMS**, as appropriate.

4 Perform a primary assessment and monitor patient's *lifeline* – **ABCD'S**.

5 Once EMS is contacted, obtain and follow local medical control directions for field treatment prior to their arrival.

6 If patient shows signs of a severe allergic reaction, treat appropriately. (See *Allergic Reactions* for more information.) Monitor the patient's *lifeline* until EMS arrives.

7 If stinger is still embedded, scrape it sideways from skin – avoid pinching or squeezing the venom sac.

8 Reassure and keep patient still and at rest.

9 Depending on the directions from EMS: a) clean the bite area with soap and water or rubbing alcohol, b) apply cold compress to area and elevate or c) apply pressure immobilization.

10 Transport to medical facility.

Patient Care – Coral, Jellyfish and Hydroid Stings

1. **STOP** – Assess and observe scene – *Is the patient still in the water? Is a venomous creature nearby?*

2. **THINK** – Consider your safety and form action plan – *How can I further protect myself and the patient?*

3. **ACT** – Check responsiveness and **ALERT** EMS, as appropriate.

4. Perform a primary assessment and monitor patient's *lifeline* – **ABCD'S**.

5. If patient shows signs of a severe allergic reaction, treat appropriately. (See *Allergic Reactions* for more information.) Monitor the patient's *lifeline* until EMS arrives.

6. Once EMS is contacted, obtain and follow local medical control directions for field treatment prior to their arrival.

7. Reassure and keep patient still and at rest.

8. Neutralize jellyfish tentacles with vinegar. Without using your bare hands, remove large tentacle fragments.

9. Apply cold compress to area. In the case of a major jellyfish sting, consider using pressure immobilization over the wound area after application of vinegar.

10. Transport to medical facility.

Patient Care – Octopus Bite and Cone Shell Sting

1. **STOP** – Assess and observe scene – *Is the patient still in the water? Is a venomous creature nearby?*

2. **THINK** – Consider your safety and form action plan – *How can I further protect myself and the patient?*

3. **ACT** – Check responsiveness and **ALERT** EMS, as appropriate.

4. Perform a primary assessment and monitor patient's *lifeline* – **ABCD'S**.

5. Once EMS is contacted, obtain and follow local medical control directions for field treatment prior to their arrival.

6. Reassure and keep patient still and at rest. Immediately place direct pressure on the wound with a sterile dressing, pad or gloved hand.

7. Apply pressure immobilization over the wound.

8. Transport to medical facility.

Patient Care – Fish Spine Injury

1. **STOP** – Assess and observe scene – *Is the patient still in the water? Is a venomous creature nearby?*

2. **THINK** – Consider your safety and form action plan – *How can I further protect myself and the patient?*

3. **ACT** – Check responsiveness and **ALERT** EMS, as appropriate.

4. Perform a primary assessment and monitor patient's *lifeline* – **ABCD'S**.

5. Once EMS is contacted, obtain and follow local medical control directions for field treatment prior to their arrival.

6. Reassure and keep patient still and at rest. Treat for shock if needed.

7. If needed, manage serious bleeding. If easily done, remove embedded fish spines.

8. Immerse wound in hot but not scalding water. Leave immersed for up to 90 minutes for pain relief. If needed repeat this treatment. If hot water does not provide pain relief, apply cold compress to the wound.

9. Clean wound with soap and water. Apply local antiseptics.

10. Seek medical assistance.

ILLNESS AND INJURY ASSESSMENT RECORD SHEET

Key Points

✔ Stop, Think, then Act.
✔ Use barriers as appropriate.
✔ Use this record sheet in the event that Emergency Medical Services (EMS) is either delayed or unavailable.
✔ As you record information on this sheet for EMS, provide measured rates per minute and descriptive terminology.

✔ To help guide your assessment, remember that:
  - The average pulse rate for adults is between 60 – 80 beats per minute.
  - Average breathing rate for adults is between 12 and 20 breaths per minute. Patient's who take less than eight breaths per minute, or more than 24 breaths per minute probably need immediate medical care.
  - Average skin temperature is warm and skin should feel dry to the touch.
  - Noticeable skin color changes may indicate heart, lung or circulation problems.

Patient Information

Name _____

☐ Male ☐ Female   Date of Birth (Day/Mon/Yr) ___ / ___ / ___   ☐ English Speaking ☐ Non-English Speaking

Address _____

State/Province _____ Country _____   City _____

☐ Medical Alert Tag? Type _____   Zip/Postal Code _____ Phone _____

Patient Condition at Beginning of Emergency Responder Care

☐ Conscious ☐ Unconscious

Patient Position Prior to Care

☐ Standing ☐ Sitting ☐ Lying

Summary – Primary and Secondary Care Provided

☐ Rescue Breathing ☐ CPR ☐ Defibrillation
☐ Serious Bleeding Management ☐ Shock Management

☐ Spinal Injury Management ☐ Conscious Choking Assistance
☐ Emergency Oxygen Use ☐ Illness Assessment ☐ Injury Assessment
☐ Bandaging ☐ Splinting
☐ Other

Patient Referred to:

☐ EMS Personnel ☐ Hospital ☐ Personal Physician ☐ None
☐ Other

© Emergency First Response, Corp., 2005

Illness Assessment

SAMPLE – Signs and Symptoms

1. How do you feel now? _____

2. What were you doing when you began to feel ill? _____

3. When did the first symptoms occur? _____

4. Where were you when the first symptoms occurred? _____

5. Patient's pulse rate _____ (use carotid or radial pulse; count beats for 30 seconds, multiply by two)

6. Describe patient's pulse: ☐ Rapid ☐ Strong ☐ Weak ☐ Slow

7. Patient's breathing is: ☐ Rapid ☐ Labored ☐ Wheezing ☐ Gasping

8. Patient complains of: ☐ Shortness of breath ☐ Chest pain ☐ Dizziness/Lightheadedness ☐ Tingling in arms/legs ☐ Numbness

9. Patient's respiration rate _____ (count respiration for 30 seconds, multiply by two; avoid telling patient you are counting respirations).

10. Has the patient been exercising? ☐ Yes ☐ No

11. Patient's skin is: ☐ Warm ☐ Hot ☐ Cool ☐ Clammy ☐ Wet ☐ Very dry

12. Color of patient's skin is: ☐ Pale ☐ Ashen (gray) ☐ Red ☐ Blue ☐ Yellowish ☐ Black and Blue Blotches

13. Dark-skinned patients, check for color changes on the nailbeds, lips, gums, tongue, palms, whites of the eyes and ear lobes:
☐ Pale ☐ Ashen (gray) ☐ Red ☐ Blue ☐ Yellowish ☐ Black and Blue Blotches

SAMPLE – Allergies

1. Is the patient allergic to any foods, drugs, airborne matter, etc.
☐ Yes ☐ No   If so, what is he/patient allergic to? _____

2. Ask the patient if he has ingested or taken anything he may be allergic to: _____
☐ Yes ☐ No

SAMPLE – Medications

1. Ask the patient: *Do you take medication?*
☐ Yes ☐ No   If yes, what type and name: _____

2. Ask the patient: *Did you take your medication today?*
☐ Yes ☐ No   How much did you take and when? _____

3. If possible, collect all medication to give to EMS personnel and/or get name of the doctor who prescribed the medication.

SAMPLE – PreExisting Medical Conditions

1. Ask the patient: *Do you have a preexisting medical condition?*
☐ Yes ☐ No   If yes, what type: _____

SAMPLE – Last Meal

1. Ask the patient: *Did you eat recently?*
☐ Yes ☐ No   If yes, what did you eat? _____

SAMPLE – Events

1. Ask the patient: *What events led up to your not feeling well?* _____

Attach additional Responder notes on separate sheet.

EMERGENCY REFERENCE

Injury Assessment

History _____

What happened? _____

How did the injury happen? _____

When did the injury occur? _____

Injury Location (Follows Injury Assessment Order. Use Injury Key to denote condition.)

☐ Head _____
☐ Ears/Nose _____
☐ Skull/Neck _____
☐ Shoulder _____
☐ Right Arm _____
☐ Right Hand _____
☐ Chest _____
☐ Abdomen _____
☐ Right Leg _____
☐ Right Foot _____

☐ Patient's Face _____
☐ Eyes _____
☐ Shoulder Blades _____
☐ Collarbones _____
☐ Left Arm _____
☐ Left Hand _____
☐ Spinal Column _____
☐ Hips _____
☐ Left Leg _____
☐ Left Foot _____

Injury Condition Key

A = Abrasion
B = Bleeding
Bu = Burns
C = Contusion (injury to tissues; no bone or skin broken)

D = Deformity
F = Fracture
L = Laceration (deep/jagged cut)
P = Pain
S = Swelling
T = Tenderness

Emergency Responder Care Given

_____
_____
_____
_____
_____
_____
_____
_____
_____

Additional Responder Notes

_____
_____
_____
_____
_____
_____